IS SHE
Naturally
Thin OR
DISCIPLINED?

BLOOMING TWIG BOOKS / NEW YORK

Always check with your doctor before beginning a new diet or exercise program, particularly if you have a medical condition or physical restrictions.

Published by:
Blooming Twig Books
PO Box 4668 # 66675
New York, NY 10163-4668
www.bloomingtwig.com

ISBN 978-1-933918-71-6
Printed in China

What People Are Saying About

Is She Naturally Thin or Disciplined?
Insider Secrets of the Sexy and Slim!

"WOW! A picture book for grown-ups! A colorful, fun, and inspiring book that shows us IT CAN BE DONE!"
~Bonnie D. Graham, TV host

"*Is She Naturally Thin, or Disciplined?* brings real women of all shapes and sizes into a wonderfully produced book with stats and photos."
~Monique Rowe, blogger

"*Is She Naturally Thin, or Disciplined?* contains a slew of fascinating weight stories from the people who are most affected by scale issues—real women. Here's to women helping other women!"
~Claudia Copquin, editor

"*Is She Naturally Thin, or Disciplined?* gives advice and tips from real women who have found a solution to their weight issues and offers motivation to those who are still finding their way. A little something for everyone!"
~Mary Jones, radio host

"This book is NOT 'another one of those'; it's radically different and inspiring. Seeing photos of women sharing their stories elevated this from another 'rah rah' book about dieting to one showing that whether you're 20 or 70, healthy weight loss and a healthy life are possible."
~Christa Allan, author

"*Is She Naturally Thin or Disciplined?* is funny and informative. I recommend it for anyone who is trying to lose weight."
~Christy Whitman, author

"*Is She Naturally Thin, or Disciplined?* is a wonderful book to read because you learn that being healthy and maintaining a fit body is a choice that requires discipline."
~Naren Arulrajah, columnist

"*Is She Naturally Thin or Disciplined? Insider Secrets of the Sexy and Slim!* is the necessary tool to help EVERYONE who wants help with body issues. This book shows us why we should 'live-it' and not 'diet' no matter how old, how fat, how thin, or how fed-up we are with our bodies."
~Jane Angelich, entrepreneur

"Whether you're naturally thin, disciplined, and/or want to shed some pounds, you'll find insight and inspiration for women of all ages within these pages. It kept me turning pages to the end!"
~Dorothy Barron, director, Parents Focused on Education

"Every woman wants to love her body and *Is She Naturally Thin, or Disciplined?* will give you the inspiration and motivation to love yours. A must-read."
~Kristin Bender, columnist

"*Is She Naturally Thin or Disciplined? Insider Secrets of the Sexy and Slim!* is a must-read for women of all ages who have weight-loss challenges, struggle with cravings, look for the magic weight-loss pill, or are obsessed with yo-yo dieting in general. This book is exactly what women need in order to start taking care of themselves and to feel and look fabulous naturally."
~Irina Wardas, www.NaturalCounselor.com

"Is She Naturally Thin or Disciplined? is the story of real women giving their insight on maintaining a healthy lifestyle and weight in age groups from the 20's through the 60's."
~Robert Medak, editor

"Anyone who has ever wondered about how to get thin will get their answers! An inspiring tome for anyone looking to lose unwanted pounds and maintain a lifetime of healthy habits, Is She Naturally Thin or Disciplined? will not disappoint!"
~Sarah Shaw, www.Entreprenette.com

"Is She Naturally Thin or Disciplined? takes a candid look into beautiful women's weight secrets. Interesting, intimate, and informative!"
~Shoshana Bennett, PhD

"Great read for all, especially us fatties! A breathe of inspiration—now where did I leave that discipline?"
~Joey Alcarese, FAB Freedom Foundation

"Is She Naturally Thin or Disciplined? Insider Secrets of the Sexy and Slim! is a must-read for any woman who wants to lose weight or simply live a healthy life. This is a book all women should have in their home libraries."
~Jennifer McDonald, blogger

"We all learn and are inspired by other women's stories, especially when they're about the universal struggle with weight. *Is She Naturally Thin or Disciplined?* can help you design your own plan for a healthy and fit lifestyle."
~Phyllis Goldberg, PhD, and Rosemary Lichtman, PhD

"If you are really interested in living a lifestyle that promotes and supports being slim, then *Is She Naturally Thin or Disciplined?* is the only book you need to read on the subject! It is a fast read, a book you will study in-depth and refer to over and over for years."
~Jackie Black, PhD

"*Is She Naturally Thin, or Disciplined?* features real women sharing their secrets to staying thin, which is much more relatable to the average woman than the thin models on the magazine covers."
~Wade Sorochan, radio host

"*Is She Naturally Thin or Disciplined? Insider Secrets of the Sexy and Slim!* is a refreshing, relatable look at the challenges of maintaining—or regaining—and embracing a healthy lifestyle. The stories are told by real women with real lives who don't have personal trainers at their beck and call, yet have made the decision to make their own health and wellness a priority"
~Denée King, www.SheJustGotMarried.com

"If you've ever had issues with self-esteem or weight, this inspiring book is perfect for you."
~Nicole Scott-Tate, www.YourChampagneWishesEvents.com

"A great book if you need a little bit of encouragement on your weight loss and/or healthy-living journey. Read brief bios of people who have been there and done it!"
~LaDonna Harris, blogger

"*Is She Naturally Thin or Disciplined? Insider Secrets of the Sexy and Slim!* is not about the 'diet' but the 'way of life.' This is a must-have book for any woman!"
~Dani Gurrie, www.Tots2Tweens.com

"This book is definitely a one-size-fits-all! Any obstacle you may have, you'll find a woman who overcame it. It's like having them do all your homework for you, from healthy living to that motivation nugget you need when you're stuck, this book is chock-full of great tips to get you toned, trim, and disciplined."
~Kelly Bouchard, success coach

"The self-discipline mentioned in *Is She Naturally Thin or Disciplined?* is like The Art of War against weight. These life stories are about more than losing weight; each is an inspirational example of true leadership. First lead yourself to a goal, then others."
~D. Miserandino, www.TheCelebrityCafe.com

"*Is She Naturally Thin or Disciplined?* Insider Secrets of the Sexy and Slim! lays out a solid plan for fighting fat and tipping the scale in your favor."
~John Basedow, TV personality and fitness DVD creator

"Sally Shields is like your BFF, giving you the best tips to get thin and stay that way. Some great advice on how to look good and feel terrific!"
~Lissa Coffey, www.CoffeyTalk.com

"Be encouraged! There are so many ways to achieve the body and lifestyle of your dreams, and *Is She Naturally Thin or Disciplined? Insider Secrets of the Sexy and Slim!* will show you exactly how!"
~Mia King, bestselling author, Sweet Life

"*Is She Naturally Thin or Disciplined?* makes you remember that beautiful women come in many shapes and sizes. Even more importantly, you'll feel like you've got a gallery of girlfriends giving you their best tips on what they really do to maintain a healthy body. It's real-world advice you can refer back to again and figure out what works for you."
~Lauren Schiller and Steph Walton, BlogTalkRadio co-hosts

IS SHE
Naturally Thin OR
DISCIPLINED?

SALLY SHIELDS

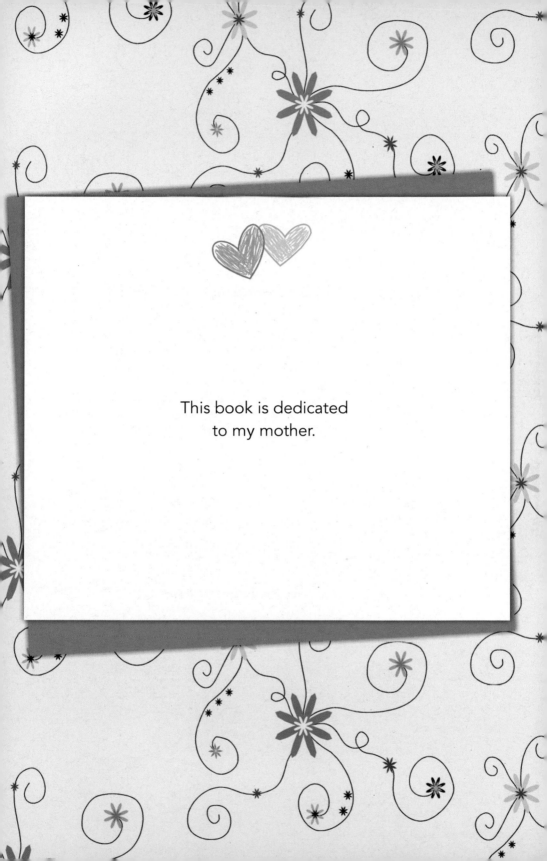

This book is dedicated
to my mother.

Contents

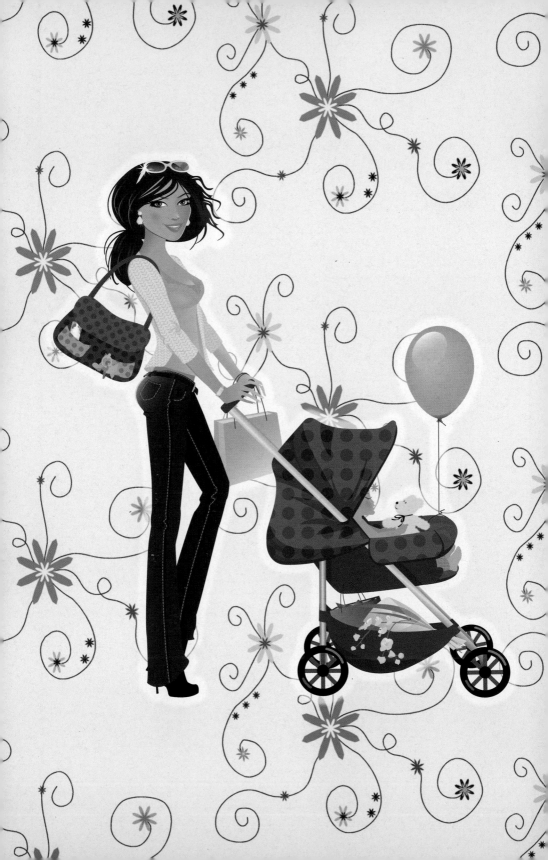

Foreword

Foreword by Victoria L. Dunckley, M.D.

"How does she stay so *thin*?"

What woman hasn't murmured that to herself upon encountering a slender member of the female species? Especially one who has had children, or is older than 30?

Even as she ponders it, behind that question is another—is it lucky genes or hard work? In this inspiring book, Sally Shields demonstrates that she again has her finger on the pulse of the collective female psyche, as 101 women share how they manage to keep fit.

I met Sally through a mutual associate; Sally had begun collecting women's stories, but had yet to embark on her own successful thin-journey. Having worked with patients on weight-loss issues and having successfully lost weight myself, I was about to walk down the aisle and wanted to help other brides achieve their dream bodies. After sharing my story with her and explaining how I believed the key was in getting a handle on biological cravings, she shared with me how she found it more difficult to even *start* losing weight, because the process is so frustrating! I decided to gift her with the five-day cleanse I'd used for myself and with my patients, in exchange for her sending some business my way.

After that, she combined a couple of different programs that worked successfully for her. For both of us (and, I assert, to all the women on these pages), success boiled down to maintaining healthy, stable blood sugar levels. This, in turn, allows us to make appropriate choices. It's when we are hungry—or worse, *ravenous*—that our bodies override our intentions in order to bring our blood sugar back up, as quickly as possible.

As I read through these 101 stories, I was struck by two things. One was the amount of planning involved in the contributors' various methods. They included grocery shopping, having healthy snacks around, and making time to exercise. This was the case even with women who said they had always been thin. Second was the number of women who were in some kind of health or nutritional field as their profession. To me, this speaks of the power of education and understanding. Maintaining one's weight is very similar to money management—building wealth does not happen by accident, and people who are "born rich" will become poor if they are careless.

> Maintaining one's weight is very similar to money management—building wealth does not happen by accident, and people who are "born rich" will become poor if they are careless.

Sally and I bonded over this experience, and her story today reinforces the notion that success is a process that starts with having *someone else* instill hope and belief. That new shared energy between two people combined with initial success and continued support, is what helps someone turn a corner.

That is why I love this book. If one person can learn one helpful nugget of information, or become encouraged in a new way, then Ms. Shields has indeed paid it forward. So read on, and get inspired!

~Victoria L. Dunckley, M.D.
www.drdunckley.com

Preface

Do you struggle with your weight? Are you the mom who perhaps gained some weight after having kids and is finding it hard to take off? Or, perchance, one who looks at super-slim women and wonders to herself whether they are naturally thin or very controlled about their diet and exercise routines?

Ever since college, I have struggled with my weight. I was obsessed with new fad diets such as calorie restriction, low-fat, low-carb, cabbage soup, Acai berry, the Zone, South Beach, and the Grapefruit, Lemonade, and Special K diets! I have fallen off the wagon and eaten pizza (many slices at one sitting) and ice cream. Whole tubs of it. Entire packages of pasta. And my personal weakness, Thai food. Lots of it.

A couple years into marriage, I experienced such hunger pangs during pregnancy that I ate on the hour, round the clock. After all, this was the proverbial time of life that one could simply eat and not be judged—a great excuse to enjoy food! Well, by the time my second child was born, I was the heaviest I'd ever been, but hey, I was a mom, right?

Nonetheless, I vowed to watch what I ate—that is, until the next hunger pang came along, and I didn't exactly feel like giving up the bagels and pasta! I thought about joining a gym, but already had an exercise bike at home, so why spend the money? So I got on it. But somehow, because I was "exercising," I also allowed myself to eat more. So when the nice lady next door came over with some holiday treats, I had three pieces. Uh-oh... The next day, I hesitantly stepped on the scale. I knew then that I had a problem, a serious problem that wasn't getting better, but in fact was getting worse. Not only was I obsessed with losing weight and dieting, but I was failing, and gaining weight. This scared me!

I wanted to lose weight, but was constantly hungry. To put it bluntly, my body wasn't budging. My mother would say, "You have two young children, give yourself a break. That's how mommies look!" But I wasn't sure that was the case entirely, as I would see other moms back to their skinny selves. I would wonder to myself if they were naturally thin, or if they were actually disciplined about their diet and exercise routines. Casually, I asked a few women how they did it. They'd tell me different things such as, "Just walk" or "Yeah, I just breast-fed, and I snapped right back!" Or it might be, "Well, I've always been thin, and I only gained 20 pounds when I was pregnant" or "If I want to lose a little weight, I just watch my carb intake for a few days and weight just falls off." I even went so far as to jokingly ask my super skinny, ribs-sticking-out, seven-year-old, gymnastics-loving daughter what her secrets were. She took my query quite seriously, and made a list that is displayed prominently on our refrigerator. It says, "How to Get Skinny, by Lara":

1. Don't eat a lot of junk food.
2. Walk up and down the stairs lots of times.
3. Do exercise bike every day.
4. Run or walk or jog places.
5. Do grown-up gymnastiks.

Very wise—diet and exercise! Of course! Why didn't I think of that?! No matter what answers I got and from whom, however, I knew in my heart that there was more to it than that. I was indeed missing some important pieces to the puzzle.

So, I thought, "Well, why not go ahead and just ask these women for their insider secrets, and not just a little piece of advice they could pass off while waiting for the kids after school." I would ask a LOT of women a LOT of questions. I would find out the real deal. I desperately wanted to be thin again! I even had a cartoon drawn of myself at my ideal weight (see the cover of this book!). Having someone sketch you thin is a lot easier than diet and exercise—LOL! But I wondered how exactly to lose weight, and keep it off, for good.

So, in typical investigative fashion, I went about gathering the myriad profiles contained in this book in order to uncover, and ultimately divulge, the secrets of the sexy and slim. I wanted to know precisely what people ate, how much, when, were they always thin, and if not, what they did about it. Did they drink a lot of water, use supplementation? What were their fitness routines, and did they include weight training? What attitudes and philosophies did they embody? And anything and everything else I could think of, I would ask them. I wanted to find out if their skinniness was a force of nature, luck of the draw, or a matter of discipline at work!

I set out to uncover some answers and to offer inspiration to those in need of a strategy. Inside this book, you will find many insider secrets to shedding those unwanted pounds once and for all, so that you can be healthy, feel fabulous, and get back into your favorite jeans again!

Candidly sharing their personal stories, these 101 contributors range from women who were born with the coveted thin gene to those who struggled to learn exactly what it takes to maintain their slim figures. So come with me on my journey to discover what it truly takes to look and feel great, no matter what your age, size or body type!

"The five S's of sports training are: stamina, speed, strength, skill, and spirit; but the greatest of these is spirit."

~Ken Doherty

The
20's

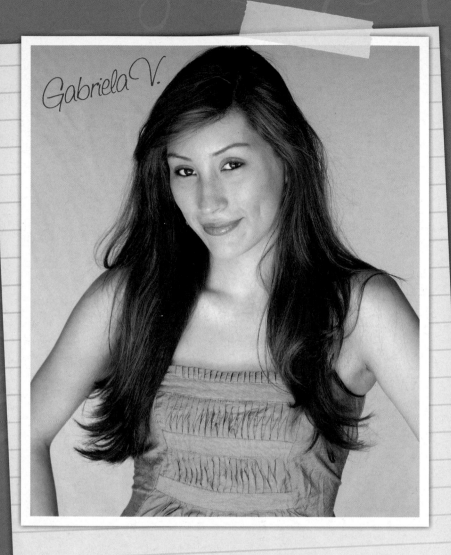

Gabriela V.

AGE:	21
HEIGHT:	5'7"
WEIGHT:	120 lbs
DRESS SIZE:	2
# OF CHILDREN:	1
PROFESSION:	actress/model

Gabriela V.

Even though I ate whatever I wanted, I remained skinny throughout childhood by keeping active with cheerleading, ballet, and swimming. But as I got older, I noticed I was getting a little flabby (especially around the middle) and I did not feel so attractive anymore. So I started to pay attention to my diet a bit more.

Today I eat a little healthier and in smaller portion sizes. I concentrate on foods that have high antioxidant value such as fresh fruits and veggies, and supplement with a women's multivitamin. And once in a while I do a little detoxification with natural teas.

For exercise, I work out on the treadmill and do some sit-ups with my Ab Lounge a little bit each day.

As long as I fuel my body with healthy foods and get a minimal amount of exercise on a daily basis, I feel healthy, attractive, and am able to maintain a body shape and size that makes me feel sexy and in tune with life!

"Today I eat a little healthier and in smaller portion sizes"

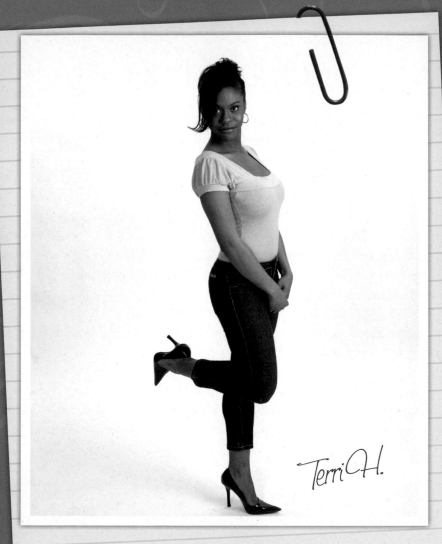

Terri H.

AGE: 21
HEIGHT: 5'0"
WEIGHT: 105 lbs
DRESS SIZE: 0
PROFESSION: writer

Terri H.

When I was four, I started ballet, and dancing continues to be a part of my life today. And even though I enjoy a naturally petite physique, I still find it of utmost importance to maintain a healthy lifestyle and diet.

Today, junk food is never an option and fruits and vegetables are essential for me with every meal. When it comes to beverages, soda is never considered. I do enjoy juice, but because of all the sugar in fruit, I stick to all-natural drinks, avoiding those that contain high-fructose corn syrup. As I get older, I appreciate the value and flavor of water much more.

I maintain an active lifestyle by following along with home workout videos a couple of times a week.

I am proud of the body that I have, and work hard to maintain it. But more than anything, I feel great when I take care of myself—by sticking to a clean, healthy diet free of processed foods and by committing to consistent and enjoyable exercise.

"junk food is never an option and fruits and vegetables are essential"

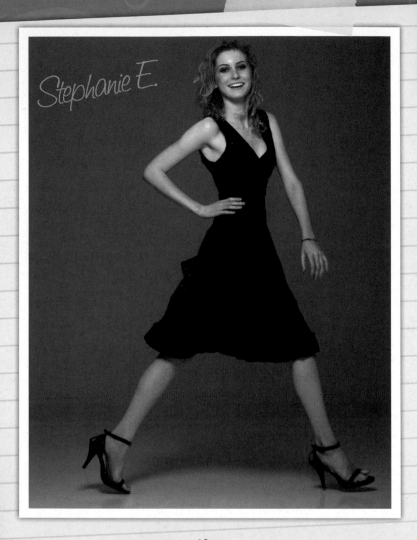

Stephanie E.

AGE: 23

HEIGHT: 5'7"

WEIGHT: 108 lbs

DRESS SIZE: 2

PROFESSION: natural skin care expert and health writer

Stephanie E.

I have always been thin. However, I consciously take measures to maintain my lean frame. For example, for me, the key to staying slender rests with four things:

1. I drink water before meals.
2. I eat four to six small portions evenly spaced out throughout the day.
3. I move my body for at least 15 minutes a day.
4. I avoid refined sugar and processed junk.

I start the day with a tall glass of water and fresh-squeezed lemon juice. Then I have breakfast, which is fruit or all-natural rice cereal with almond milk. I eat every two hours or so thereafter, sticking to small portions. I mainly enjoy plant-based meals such as brown rice, steamed veggies, and fresh organic fruit. But if I do eat animal products, I make sure there are no added hormones or antibiotics. I love raw honey as a sweetener, but avoid refined sugar such as what you'll find in white bread, pasta, and high-fructose corn syrup. I supplement with fish oil, vitamin C powder, lutein for antioxidant protection, and Epic Elixirs' Elixir of Immortality honey herb blend.

I exercise every day for a minimum of 30 minutes a day. I do yoga, Pilates, and follow Zuzana Light's circuit training routines with her home workout videos.

It takes a conscious effort to maintain a daily habit of exercise. I don't always want to do it, but I love the results and always feel better afterwards. There is something about the endorphins that get released from exercise that makes me feel absolutely positive about going about the rest of my day. To me, that feeling alone is worth the effort!

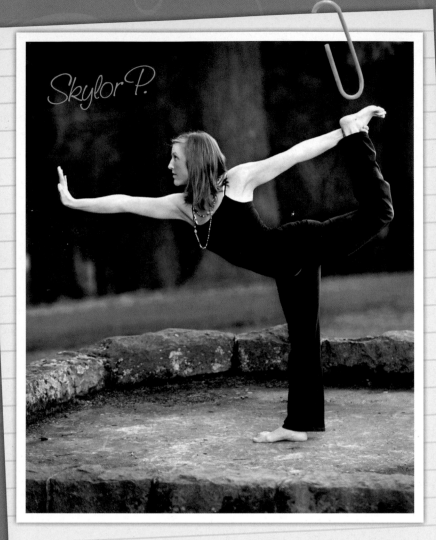

Skylor P.

AGE:	23
HEIGHT:	5'1"
WEIGHT:	107 lbs
DRESS SIZE:	2
PROFESSION:	yoga instructor, holistic health counselor

Skylor P.

Growing up I was a lot heavier than I needed to be for my diminutive stature. Therefore, I began exercising and replacing processed foods with things that actually come from the earth! As a result, my weight dropped and I'm now able to maintain a comfortable and well-proportioned body.

Today I eat three meals a day that are packed with protein and vegetables. Greens such as spinach, kale, arugula, broccoli, or chard are common components in my diet as well as grains such as quinoa, buckwheat and brown rice. What don't I eat? Sugar, white bread, and high-fructose corn syrup are three things I never put into my body! I also pay attention to how food makes me feel. For example, if something upsets my stomach or makes me tired, then I avoid it in the future. I supplement with bee pollen and an Omega-3 daily.

My exercise routine involves yoga a few times a week. I also make a point of walking or biking if my destination is close.

In order to get through the day with energy and enthusiasm, I want my body as healthy as it can be. Therefore, I stick to a diet high in protein and vegetables, do not overeat, and exercise for about an hour a day. And rather than being concerned with the scale, I think more about my overall energy level and daily activity commitment. As a result, my weight stays balanced and I am a happier person!

"I also make a point of walking or biking if my destination is close."

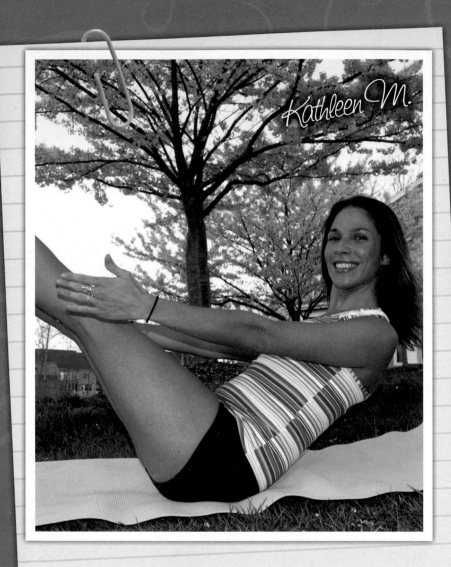

Kathleen M.

AGE:	24
HEIGHT:	5'8"
WEIGHT:	125 lbs
DRESS SIZE:	2
PROFESSION:	public relations professional

Kathleen M.

I was the heavy girl growing up and disliked any kind of exercise. I would often fake a headache and purposely forget my sneakers on gym day. And when my friends were involved in afterschool sports, I was home watching Oprah! When I headed to college, my mother teased that I should watch out for weight gain. At that moment, I decided not only was I going to avoid the freshman 15, but I also I was going to lose some! So, I went to the gym, got on the treadmill, and did some weight training a few times a week. Before I knew it, I was in the best shape of my life! I also changed my relationship with food.

Today, I eat four to six small meals a day and always have on-the-go energy snacks on hand. I stock my fridge with clean, whole foods such as fruits, vegetables, dairy, nuts, and lean proteins. Some of my staple meals and snacks include eggs on a whole-wheat wrap with avocado and salsa, yogurt with honey and walnuts, and chicken spinach salad with balsamic vinaigrette. I also keep a tub of vanilla-flavored protein powder in my house to mix into smoothies, oatmeal, and even baked goods to help satisfy cravings.

I work out five to six days a week, alternating training with free weights, total conditioning classes, Pilates, and plyometrics. When I hit a plateau or a slump in motivation I makeover my iPod playlist, turn to my favorite fitness magazines to get creative on how to spice up my routines and get new clean meal ideas, or even treat myself to a new gym outfit to help bust out of my rut.

I approach an active lifestyle as my biggest investment in myself. When it comes to my body, I have conditioned myself to own it, respect it, and provide it with the energy it needs so that I can be my best self.

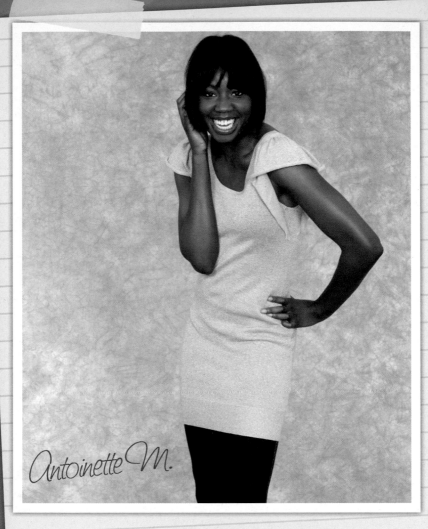

Antoinette M.

AGE:	24
HEIGHT:	5'9"
WEIGHT:	130 lbs
DRESS SIZE:	4
PROFESSION:	writer, model, creator of an online magazine for entrepreneurs

Antoinette M.

I have the genetic composition of tall and thin, but thin does not always equal healthy! Most people learn about words like riboflavin, folic acid, and antioxidants when they read labels when food shopping, but I was taught what these meant at a very young age. And as I have always been fond of veggies and fruits, to this day, sugary snacks are totally out of the question.

Today with my unpredictable schedule, it is often challenging to fit in a well-balanced breakfast, but a banana or yogurt carries me over to the next meal quite well. For lunch you can find me building a savory and filling salad at Hale and Hearty. By dinner I revert to fish or baked chicken with a side salad. Every now and then I'll splurge on a greasy meal such as pizza or Chinese, but I feel sluggish afterwards so I usually wait a couple of weeks between guilty pleasures. I also avoid fried foods and soda, which are only allowed in my house during the holidays. And to keep my body flushed of toxins, I drink at least six bottles of water a day.

As a model, measurements are everything, and a low number on the scale does not necessarily omit the unattractive bulge lingering around the midsection! Therefore, I aggressively walk for 15 minutes each morning, and again at the end of the day for an additional 30 minutes. I also do floor exercises to maintain my slender frame and strive for that flat-belly look.

For me, portion control and significant activity are the keys to enjoying a healthy mind, body, and spirit.

"To keep my body flushed of toxins, I drink at least six bottles of water a day."

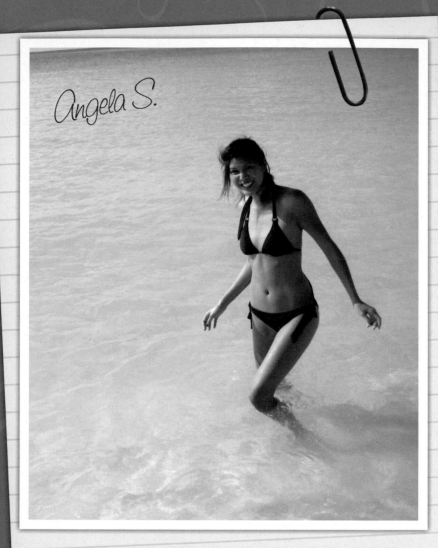

Angela S.

AGE:	25
HEIGHT:	5'5"
WEIGHT:	105 lbs
DRESS SIZE:	0
PROFESSION:	registered dietitian

Angela S.

I used to be a "do as I say, not as I do" type of gal. For example, I would eat fried foods and enjoy drinks after a day at work counseling patients on high cholesterol. It wasn't until I experienced a significant weight gain that I started to practice what I preached!

Today I eat four to five times a day, and include at least 30 grams of fiber by having steel-cut oats for breakfast and vegetables with lunch and dinner. I aim for a diet high in monounsaturated fat (I eat pistachios) and low in saturated fat (I avoid red meat). Staples include nonfat yogurt, light cheese, whole-wheat crackers, and apples with natural peanut butter. I don't believe in drinking calories so I avoid juice, soda, and anything with a sugar substitute. I supplement with folic acid and vitamin D along with a daily multivitamin.

I'm at the gym five times a week for a total of six to eight hours a week. My workouts include yoga, Pilates, and either a definitions or a step class.

A combination of clean, healthy eating and moderate, consistent exercise keeps me feeling healthy and energetic. It's hard work and takes a big commitment to stick with it, but exercise and eating well have become habit-forming. I see a high quality of life in my future as a result of my conscientious choices today!

"I avoid juice, soda, and anything with a sugar substitute"

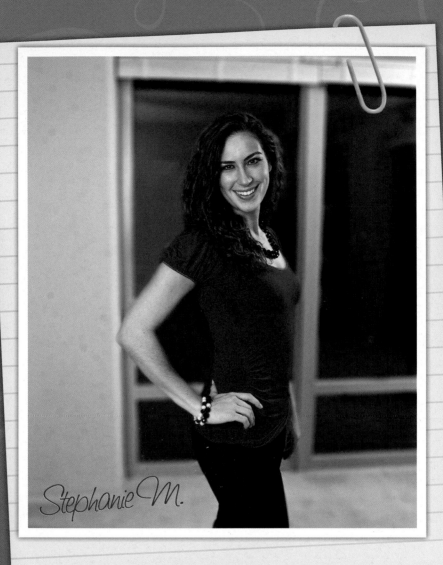

Stephanie M.

AGE:	25
HEIGHT:	5'7"
WEIGHT	145 lbs
DRESS SIZE:	4
PROFESSION:	health and fitness expert, body image and confidence coach

Stephanie M.

I n high school I played team sports, worked out, and kept to a pretty healthy diet. However, all my good eating habits went out the window when I got to college, where I found myself indulging in junk food. The result? I gained a bit more than the freshman 15, to sum it up! I eventually learned that blood sugar levels need to remain constant in order to combat cravings for sugar and simple carbs. I eventually accomplished this by eating protein every few hours, and in an effort to regain my figure, I started going to the gym.

I have become quite in-tune with how my body feels after eating certain things as I notice getting lethargic after indulging in a donut or bag of chips. Therefore, I am now all about eating pure, whole foods, and steering clear of anything with ingredients I can't pronounce. I eat five times a day, including protein and a fruit or vegetable at each meal. Some examples are a whey protein smoothie, salad with beans, gluten-free pasta with chicken, stir-fried veggies and brown rice, and scrambled eggs with avocado and apple slices, to name a few.

I maintain a yoga practice along with light weight lifting and about ten minutes of interval cardio training a few times a week.

I attribute my overall health to positive change in my dietary practices as well as the effectiveness of my workouts. I look forward to the future, having confidence in the ability to maintain my health, energy levels, and capacity to slow down the aging process by paying attention to correct habits each and every day.

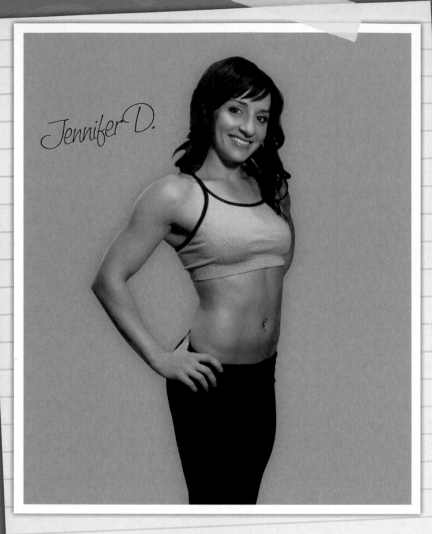

Jennifer D.

AGE:	27
HEIGHT:	4'11"
WEIGHT:	110 lbs
DRESS SIZE:	2
PROFESSION:	personal fitness trainer, business owner

Jennifer D.

G rowing up I was encouraged to play sports. Although I still love health and fitness, there are certainly days when I'd rather sleep than hit the gym! But what keeps me going is knowing that my body will thank me for following through with my healthy habits!

Although exercise is a must for maintaining a healthy, toned body, I've found that nutrition accounts for most of the results I get, so I am conscious of everything I eat. I consume five to six small meals a day including lean protein such as egg whites, and healthy fats from almonds or peanut butter. I have as many vegetables as possible, staying away from high-sugar foods and white carbs like the plague. Fruit and natural sugars are also things I am careful with because sugar is still sugar, and I make a point to skip the bread at restaurants. I supplement with a multivitamin, calcium, glutamine, and vitamin C daily.

To manage and maintain my optimum body, I set the alarm each morning and get my workout out of the way. I exercise about an hour six days a week and as a result, it no longer feels like a chore (at least on most days!).

I don't focus on the scale or the size of my jeans; rather, I concentrate on the accomplishment of my workouts, getting enough rest and taking the correct supplements. My slogan is, "Fit bodies don't just happen, they're made!" I have learned that the secret to my success is to enjoy what I do. And that's especially true in a fitness plan!

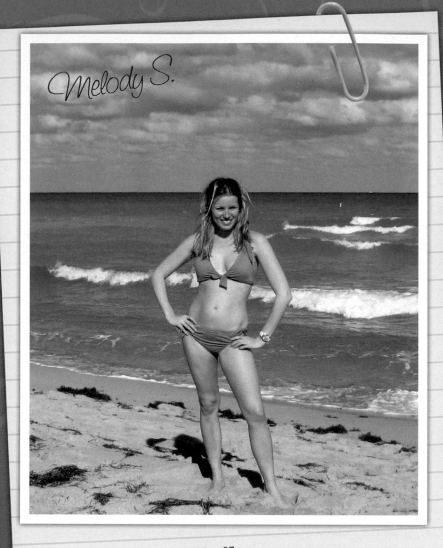

Melody S.

AGE: 27

HEIGHT: 5'2"

WEIGHT: 106 lbs

DRESS SIZE: 1

PROFESSION: communication director, writer

Melody S.

When I was young, I was downright skinny. I could gobble up a plate of greasy fries and an ice cream sundae and never see the consequences. However, when I reached college, all that started to change, and well, frankly, that frightened me! So I took stock, made some adjustments, and my weight began to stabilize.

Today I maintain a vegetarian diet. I eat breakfast, lunch, and dinner with small, healthy snacks between meals. I don't read labels or think about calories, but I do watch what I eat. For example, you won't catch me chugging soda or munching on potato chips. But I don't want to be tempted either, so I make a point of keeping unhealthy snacks out of my cabinets. However, every so often I'll indulge a bit, sure, but for me, moderation is key.

I work out five to six times a week, switching up my workouts between walking, running, spin class, dancing, the elliptical machine, abdominal exercises, and weight training. I can sense when my fitness routines are working and tightening my muscles, which feels great! But I also feel the fatigue set in if I skip too many days in a row, so that is enough motivation to keep me on track.

I don't worry much about my weight, remaining only mildly aware of the number on the scale. But the key combination of an active lifestyle coupled with a healthy eating philosophy allows me to stay fit and feel great!

"Every so often I'll indulge a bit, sure, but for me, moderation is key."

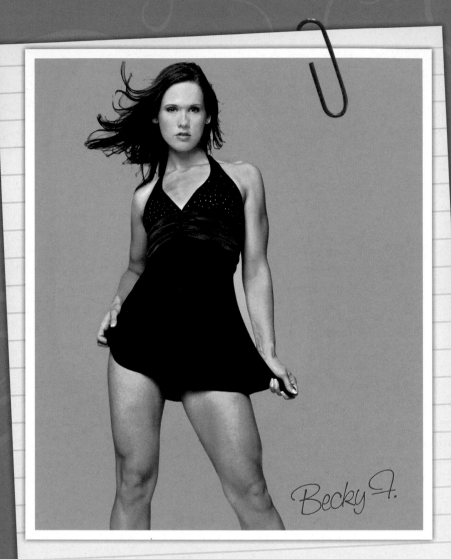

Becky T.

AGE:	27
HEIGHT:	5'9"
WEIGHT:	138 lbs
DRESS SIZE:	8
PROFESSION:	personal trainer, model

Becky F.

Growing up everyone called me a beanstalk. But when I reached my senior year, I decided I wanted curves, so I made some small changes like drinking more water and going to the gym to lift weights. Before long, I started getting the results I was looking for, and that just gave me the incentive to keep going!

Today I eat every two to three hours for a total of five to six times per day. I do this to keep the metabolism up and help my body maintain that hard-earned muscle. It also stabilizes my blood sugar, keeps energy levels high, and prevents hunger so I'm not tempted to binge and eat anything in sight! I also like counting calories, so I aim for about 300–350 calories per meal. Breakfast includes egg whites with spinach, peppers, and onions, or oatmeal sweetened with stevia and berries, followed by a protein shake for a mid-morning snack. I love sweet potatoes with cinnamon, so I have this with a lean protein and salad for lunch. Mid-afternoon I have another protein shake with some fruit and raw almonds. For dinner, I have a lean protein and veggies such as green beans or broccoli with a small side of brown rice or quinoa. I drink water nonstop, so you'll rarely see me without one of those 24-ounce stainless steel water bottles in hand! I stay away from fried, fast, and junk food, avoid artificial sweeteners, and limit dairy products. I may have a cheat-meal once a week or so, but I keep that very limited. I supplement with protein powder and glutamine to aid in recovery and muscle growth.

I work with weights about three to four times a week, focusing on a different body part each time, such as shoulders, arms, chest, legs, and back. I throw in abdominal exercises a couple of times a week as well. As for cardio, I do intervals on the treadmill or elliptical, jump rope, or take a spin class. And in nice weather, I get outdoors to run or bike.

Maintaining a healthy physique makes me feel good and gives me energy. I have developed a set of lifestyle changes that I can stick with for the long haul, and have ended up loving the consequences!

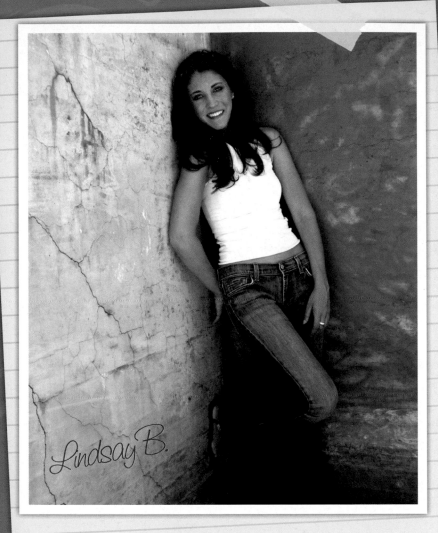

Lindsay B.

AGE:	28
HEIGHT:	5'7"
WEIGHT:	115 lbs
DRESS SIZE:	0
PROFESSION:	registered dietitian

Lindsay B.

I always had a pretty small frame. Even so, I live by the "everything in moderation" rule—that is, eating healthy most of the time with the occasional indulgence. I stick to three meals a day and an afternoon snack. Breakfast is oatmeal with walnuts and yogurt, lunch is a peanut butter and jelly sandwich, baby carrots and fruit, and dinner is a lean protein with a sweet potato and steamed veggies. I do *not* keep chips, cookies, and ice cream in the house! And when I go out to eat, I look at the dessert menu first and plan my meal accordingly. And as I prefer to eat my calories rather than drink them, I opt for water over soda, juice, or sugary teas.

My exercise regimen is basically two to three 10- to 15-minute walks with my dog daily. Additionally, I do yoga and resistance bands and/or light weights for muscle toning.

The scale is not something I pay close attention to. Rather, a combination of eating well, moderate exercise, and an overall philosophy of health allow me to maintain my slender frame and feel good about my well being, now and in the future!

"I live by the "everything in moderation" rule"

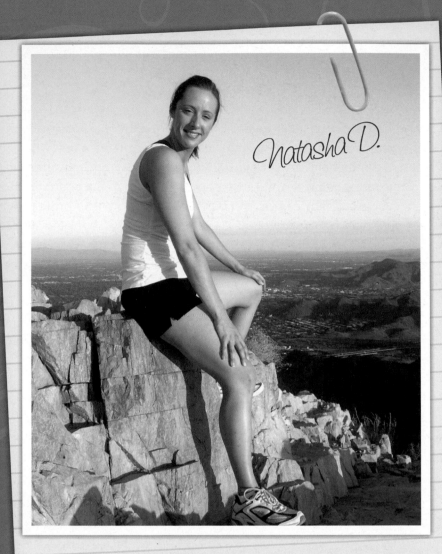

Natasha D.

AGE: 28

HEIGHT: 5'5"

WEIGHT: 125 lbs

DRESS SIZE: 2/4

OF CHILDREN: 2

PROFESSION: business development
strategist, mom

Natasha D.

Lifting weights and cardio was a weekly routine throughout high school and college, so I ate what I wanted and never gained a pound. However, after giving birth I didn't have time or energy to hit the gym and at 185 pounds, found myself extremely overweight for the first time in my life. During this time, I had developed a daily Starbucks habit and on one occasion asked how many calories were in the oat fudge bar I had just ordered. I was horrified to learn that it packed a whopping 465 calories. Add a latte and I was consuming nearly 900 calories FOR A SNACK! I knew I had to change my habits if I was going to lose weight, so I started a food journal. Writing down what I ate made my goals more tangible and helped me find the willpower to resist temptations. And as I got more fit, I craved healthier foods and looked for inventive ways to integrate them into my diet.

Today I eat five to six small meals a day. I have a healthy smoothie every morning, make fun wraps instead of just salad, and stay away from all things processed. I also drink plenty of water.

Although I worked out five times a week to lose the original weight, I now maintain my thin frame by working out three times a week. I often go with a friend, to keep me consistent and have someone other than myself to be accountable.

Keeping a food journal, finding a workout buddy, making smart food choices, and counting calories are the keys to my success. I now have the energy I need to take care of my family, and I'm able to easily maintain a body that I can be proud of!

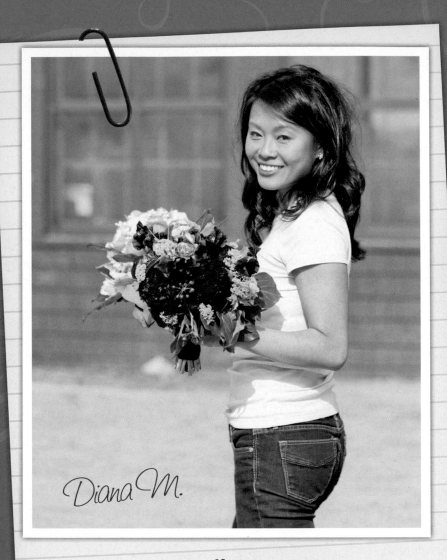

Diana M.

AGE:	29
HEIGHT:	5'1"
WEIGHT:	100 lbs
DRESS SIZE:	0
PROFESSION:	wedding professional

Diana M.

Growing up I was encouraged to stop eating as soon as I felt full. So today as an adult, if there is still food on my plate, I don't feel the need to finish it. I naturally tune into my internal clock when satisfied and turn to something else for comfort or stress relief.

I make a point to have at least one non-rushed meal a day. I really enjoy my meals and love creating all sorts of dishes—everything from pasta and veggie stir-frys to grilling and baking. I supplement with a multivitamin daily.

Exercise helps clear my head and keep my energy levels up. If it's a nice day, I run. Otherwise, I spend five to six days a week at the gym circuit training. And I'm always sure to have plenty of water during my workouts.

To me, being healthy in mind, body, and spirit keeps me feeling great. I stay grateful, do what I love, and surround myself with supportive, nurturing people. When I do this, I exude an inner confidence and radiate beauty!

"I make a point to have at least one non-rushed meal a day."

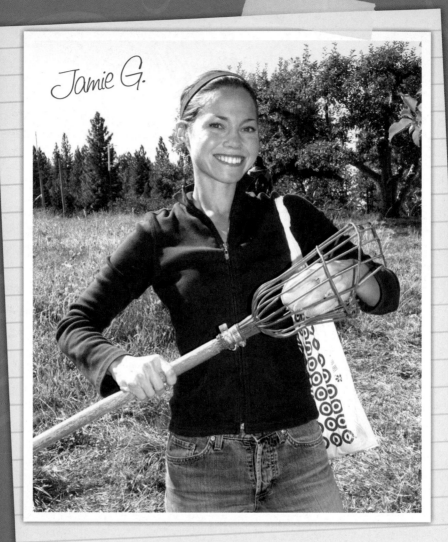

Jamie G.

AGE: 29

HEIGHT: 5'3"

WEIGHT: 110 lbs

DRESS SIZE: 2

PROFESSION: web site designer

Jamie G.

In high school, between studying overtime and not being so athletic, I gained weight continually until senior year. Then I fell in love. Incredibly nervous, I could hardly eat, and in one month, I dropped most of the weight! At first I was concerned about my lack of appetite; then I just worried about putting the pounds back on. College brought new challenges: questionable cafeteria fare and ubiquitous junk food. To my dismay, I started gaining weight again, even with my hearty walks around campus. Terrified, I got onto a treadmill. With something akin to wonder, I realized that I could run an entire mile—an act I had *never* been able to accomplish during gym class in high school! And when I realized the amount of sugar in soft drinks, I switched to drinking water and made sure to have five to ten large glasses a day.

I now pay close attention to my diet. Breakfast is a quarter cup of granola with a banana and raisins. Lunch is a sandwich with meat, lettuce, and yogurt instead of mayo. For dinner I have a large mixed salad followed by anything from roast beef and potatoes to sautéed fish. I only have one rule: to never go back for seconds.

Running is still my exercise of choice, and I do about three miles a few times a week.

My focus is less about caloric intake and more about avoiding processed foods and getting regular exercise. As a result of the healthy choices I make, I notice a direct and distinct correlation between what I eat and how much energy I have. I have learned that when treating my body well, I just feel better! This gives me the incentive to stay the path and look forward to the future with confidence!

"Physical fitness is not only one of
the most important keys to a healthy body,
it is the basis of dynamic and
creative intellectual activity."

~John Fitzgerald Kennedy

The 30's

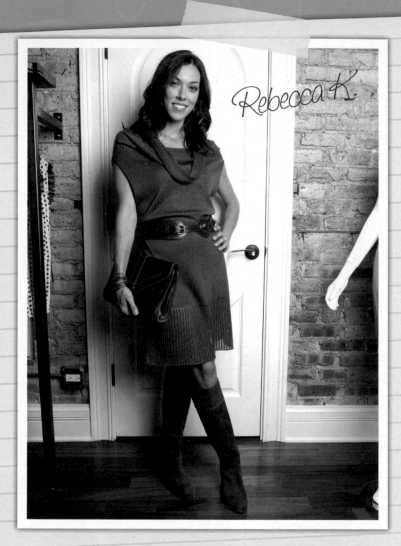

Rebecca K.

AGE:	30
HEIGHT:	5'7"
WEIGHT:	127 lbs
DRESS SIZE:	2/4
PROFESSION:	publicist

Rebecca K.

I was thin growing up and could enjoy whatever foods I wanted. But as a teen, I started gaining weight and realized I had to pay attention to my diet and start exercising.

Today I eat every couple hours. I have oatmeal for breakfast, followed by a mid-morning snack such as a protein bar, almonds, unsalted pretzels, low-fat yogurt, cheese sticks, carrots, or fruit. I avoid milk, bread, and high-fat nuts such as cashews and walnuts, as well as packaged, processed, frozen, and fast foods. I have a sensible dinner, which includes lean protein and vegetables, and I practice portion control by consuming one serving size. I drink eight glasses of water a day, avoiding soda and juice. I supplement with fish oil, flaxseed oil, Ginkgo Biloba, calcium, and antioxidants such as A, B, C, D and E.

I exercise at home with DVDs four to five times a week. I do Turbo Jam, Brazil Butt Lift (which tones my butt, hips, and thighs), Tae-Bo, and The Firm.

I think about my weight constantly, but for me it's more about being healthy and making sure my diet is clean and that I get enough exercise. Overall, these good choices help me with fatigue and mood elevation, and keep me motivated to improve other areas of my life as well.

"I exercise at home with DVDs four to five times a week."

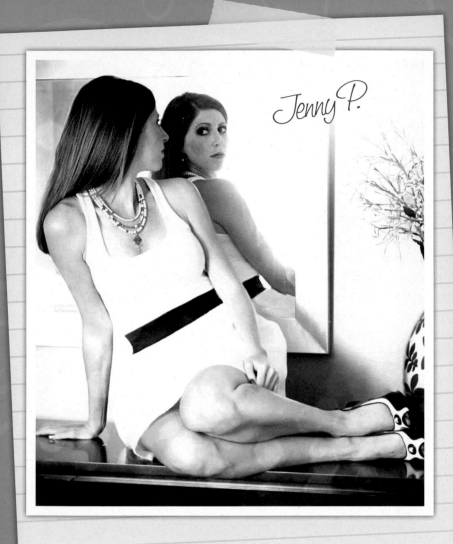

Jenny P.

AGE:	30
HEIGHT:	5'6"
WEIGHT:	105 lbs
DRESS SIZE:	0
# OF CHILDREN:	1
PROFESSION:	jewelry designer

Jenny P.

I have been a vegetarian most of my life and feel that, as a result, I have been successful in maintaining my weight.

I start the day with low-fat organic yogurt, seasonal berries, and cheerios or grape nuts mixed in. Lunch is often a salad—something I can make quickly with field greens, avocado, strawberries, feta, and balsamic vinaigrette. Dinner includes a meatless product such as un-chicken nuggets and spicy black bean burgers from Morningstar Farms®. When shopping, I buy low-fat and organic whenever possible, read labels, and stay away from anything containing high-fructose corn syrup. I don't snack, but I do have a bit of a sweet tooth. For me, moderation is key; I eat what tastes good, such as a delicious cookie—just one cookie, that is, not the whole box!

To stay active, I run. When I first started, I couldn't even go ten minutes without stopping! But now I make sure to keep going for at least 40 minutes, and I always feel great afterwards.

Living a healthy and active lifestyle are key components to my overall wellness and peace of mind!

"I have been a vegetarian most of my life"

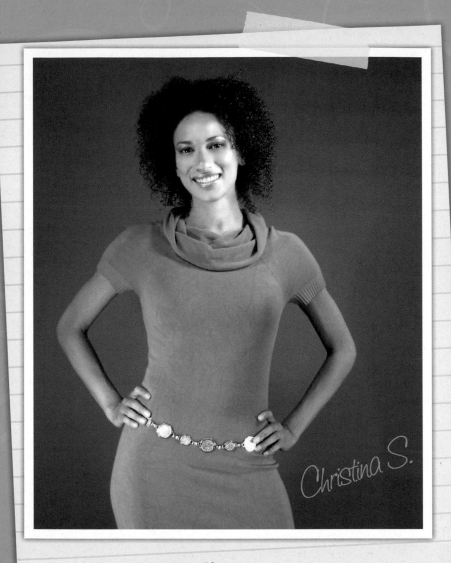

Christina S.

AGE:	30
HEIGHT:	5'10"
WEIGHT:	130 lbs
DRESS SIZE:	4
PROFESSION:	pilot, philanthropist, and personal finance expert

Christina S.

I come from a family of football players, and to this day I eat like a 12-year-old boy! So I put together a few rules to live by that help me maintain my figure, despite my sizeable appetite. And those things are:

- I listen to my body. If I am hungry, I eat, and if I'm thirsty, I drink.
- I drink a minimum of six to eight cups of water and/or tea a day.
- I don't drink soda.
- I don't eat fast food.
- I don't take diet pills.
- I don't eat cheese out of a can, bottle, or in powdered form.
- I avoid the microwave.
- I don't eat iceberg lettuce, instead sticking to dark, leafy greens like spinach or endive.
- I eat dark chocolate as it is a natural antidepressant, good for the heart, releases endorphins, and lowers cholesterol.
- I detoxify by pumping myself full of super-foods. It's kind of like hitting the reset button on my colon.
- I drink red wine. It is good for my heart and blood, and is high in antioxidants.
- I don't count calories. I just make sure I burn them off.
- I stay active by dancing, walking in nature, and doing yoga.
- I bounce. The trampoline is good for muscles, joints, lymphatic system, blood, heart, and brain!
- I stay young and happy by having fun and maintaining a positive outlook on life.

The combination of the above keeps me slim, happy, and in healthy form. I grew up enjoying meals, and have found a way to incorporate a love of food into a lifestyle that I can live with without feeling deprived. As a result, I end up getting the best of both worlds—loving to eat and a trim body to boot!

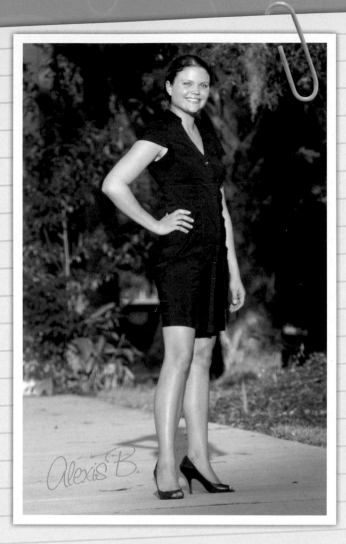

Alexis B.

AGE: 30

HEIGHT: 5'4"

WEIGHT 120 lbs

DRESS SIZE: 2

PROFESSION: public relations and brand management professional

Alexis B.

Growing up I learned that health and appearance are crucial components to achieving positive results in any endeavor. So natural foods, whole-body habits, and healthy weight maintenance have become my most successful lifestyle regimens.

Today my diet is rich in healthy fats, fruits, and vegetables. For breakfast I include whole grains and fruit, which keeps me energetic until lunch, at which point I have a salad with plenty of vegetables. I incorporate healthy snacks, such as fruit and nuts, throughout the day to boost my metabolism and curb hunger. For dinner I stick to lean protein and veggies. I drink eight to ten cups of water per day, completely avoiding soda or drinks sweetened with sugar. I supplement with Resveratrol (from Reserveage Organics) to support cardiovascular health while increasing endurance for workouts. I also take a collagen booster that moisturizes and supports skin tone and elasticity, and a multivitamin that provides a daily dose of vitamins and minerals.

I exercise several times per week, focusing on walking, dance, yoga, and Pilates.

I rarely step on a scale, but I have seen changes in my body as I mature. So by integrating the above core values into my daily routines, I am able to successfully maintain my weight as well as experience positive outcomes in many other areas of my life.

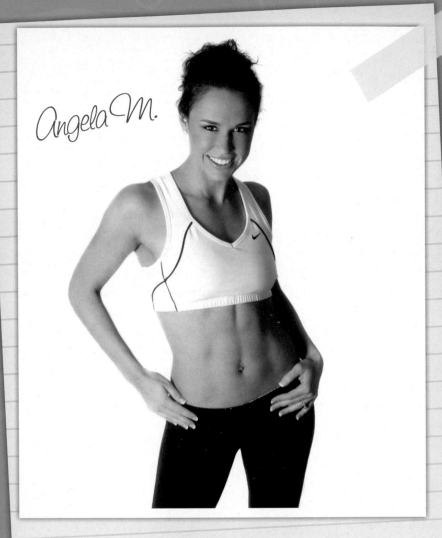

Angela M.

AGE:	30
HEIGHT:	5'2"
WEIGHT:	115 lbs
DRESS SIZE:	2
PROFESSION:	entrepreneur, health enthusiast, author

Angela M.

My secret to being healthy and fit is keeping a workout and food log. Planning my weekly workouts on Sunday night gets me motivated and ensures that I schedule exercise into my day versus trying to find time. And logging my food makes me think twice about eating something that I may not want to write down.

I start the day with either oatmeal or protein pancakes. Lunch is a big spinach salad with protein and quinoa or brown rice, and my afternoon snack is an apple with a handful of almonds or Greek yogurt and berries. For dinner I stick to lean protein and veggies. Depending on when my workout is, I'll have a protein shake right before to fuel my body and plan to have a meal right after the workout. When I do go out to eat, I skip the bread and share dessert. Once a week I treat myself to frozen yogurt, which I enjoy post-workout when my body can process sugar the fastest, and it actually repairs muscle by replacing glucose. I drink eight to ten glasses of water a day because it provides me with a full feeling, and as a result, I end up eating less. And my one rule: no eating after 9 p.m.—lights out!

I do strength training and cardio five to six days a week. Lifting usually lasts 30 minutes and I always circuit each set with cardiovascular or abdominal exercises in between to keep my heart rate up. Cardio usually includes two days on either the Stairmaster or elliptical for 30–40 minutes, a group exercise class, and then spinning, running, or Pilates once a week. My favorite workout is boot-camp style at the beach where I run in the sand, do lunges up and down some stairs, and push-ups in the grass. It's tough, but leaves me feeling refreshed. Even on my off-days I go for a walk, as I just feel better both physically and mentally when I move my body.

Living a fit and healthy life is my passion, but that doesn't mean it comes easy. Every day I make the decision to challenge myself physically as well as choose healthy foods to fuel my body. As a result, I enjoy the way I look and feel—and end up having great energy every day!

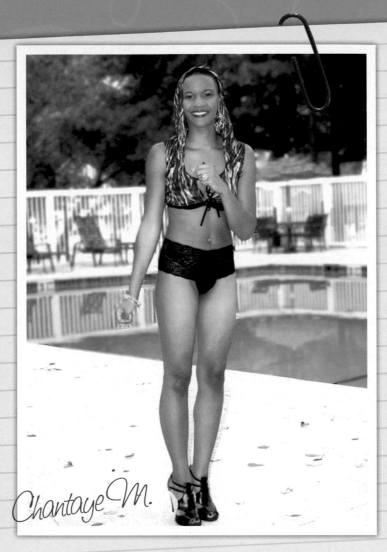

Chantaye M.

AGE: 30

HEIGHT: 5'7"

WEIGHT: 120 lbs

DRESS SIZE: 2/4

 # OF CHILDREN: 1

PROFESSION: public relations, marketing and finance expert, speaker, writer, humanitarian

Chantaye M.

I have always had a thin frame. However, thin does not always equal healthy! The positive changes I made in my diet were more about my desire for clear skin and overall health than size.

Today, I eat several times a day, preferring fresh and organic produce to anything frozen or processed. And when preparing vegetables, I add seasoning to maintain their nutritional value. I do not eat red meat or anything out of a box or can. I kicked my soda habit and replaced it with tea (no sugar). I also drink a lot of water, which rids the body of impurities as well as aides with an overall feeling of hydration and wellness.

Although the bulk of my activity consists of chasing around a four-year-old and dodging flying toys, I take long walks with the dog each morning. And if I feel the need to tone, I do yoga or something fun like indoor rock climbing, and my stomach gets totally tight. I also love to dance.

The combination of doing what I love in life, finding ways to exercise that are pleasurable, and making healthy dietary choices keep me staying slim and feeling great!

"I take long walks with the dog each morning"

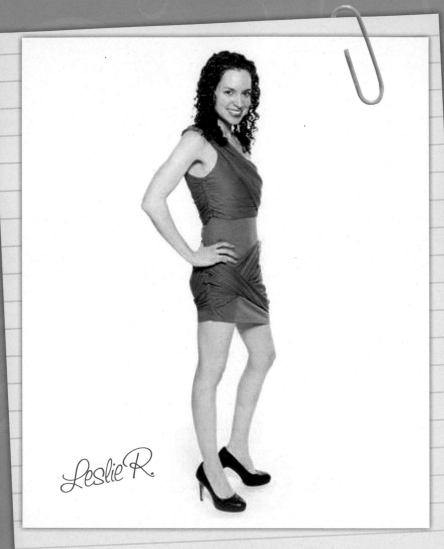

Leslie R.

AGE:	32
HEIGHT:	5'3"
WEIGHT:	90 lbs
DRESS SIZE:	0
PROFESSION:	freelance journalist, publicist, social media strategist, event planner

Leslie R.

When I was a teen, people often inquired about my weight and asked if I "broke" easily. As an adult, I continue to receive comments about my petite frame; however, I love to eat and do so quite often. Although I have a naturally slim physique, I am mindful about what I put into my body because I want to maintain my health, now and in the future.

I enjoy an iced soy chai tea for breakfast, and eat a salad, sandwich, or sushi for lunch. For dinner I stick to vegetables, whole-wheat pasta and fish, but I won't pass on dessert. I take a multivitamin and drink water throughout the day. What I don't do is smoke, drink soda or alcohol, or keep sweets in my apartment.

I exercise two to three times a week, my staples being yoga, weight training, and speed walking.

I may be thin, but I am extremely healthy and continue to live by the principles that work for me and my body. I can't actually remember the last time I caught a cold or took a sick day. For me, being in good physical condition really does come down to paying attention to my body's needs, eating well, and getting enough exercise to maintain a healthy weight.

"I take a multivitamin and drink water throughout the day."

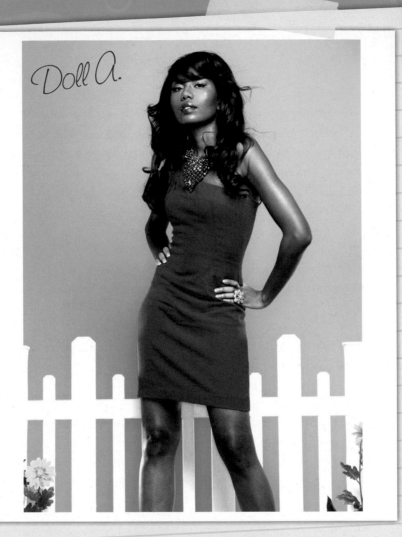

Doll A.

AGE:	32
HEIGHT:	5'9"
WEIGHT:	125 lbs
DRESS SIZE:	2
# OF CHILDREN:	2
PROFESSION:	performer, singer, songwriter, actress, musician

Doll A.

Although I am—and have always been—thin, I am careful to eat both healthily and consistently, so I can maintain a good, physically strong body.

I always have breakfast, even if it's only a granola bar or a piece of fruit. I eat every three to four hours thereafter or I run out of energy! I love fresh fruit and salad, and make sure to get enough protein throughout the day. I avoid dairy, but I do have a sweet tooth, so if someone offers me a cookie, I'll have one. But I'm just as happy eating raw carrots and broccoli. I also drink water throughout the day, which keeps my skin glowing and helps aid with proper digestion.

As far as exercise goes, I jog three to four days a week.

To sum it up, following good habits helps me to stay healthy and energetic every day!

"I eat every three to four hours thereafter or I run out of energy"

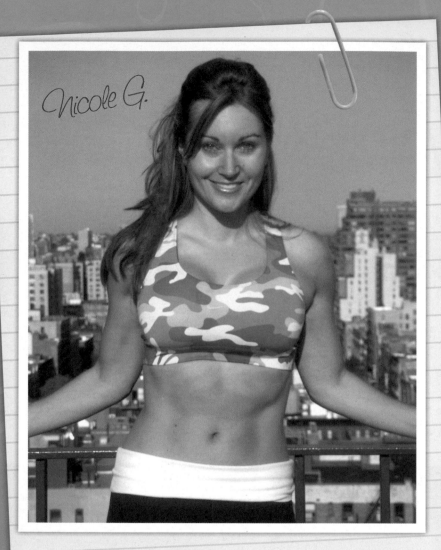

Nicole G.

AGE:	33
HEIGHT:	5'2"
WEIGHT:	103 lbs
DRESS SIZE:	2
# OF CHILDREN:	1
PROFESSION:	fitness trainer, fitness DVD creator, columnist

Nicole G.

I was active throughout high school, and when I got to college I joined the cheerleading team so I kept in shape and it was fun. However, after graduation, work, winter weather, motherhood, and metabolism set in. So in order to maintain my figure, I discovered to my horror that I really had to work at it!

Today I eat six small meals a day and never let myself get famished, because that is when I make bad food choices. My diet consists of lean protein, fruits and veggies, and only carbs that are of the whole-wheat variety. I love Fiber One® products and apples for that flat-belly look, and drink a ton of water by filling up a cute pitcher and making sure it gets emptied by nightfall. I avoid processed foods at all costs.

I take at least two cardio/sculpting classes each week. I like multitasking my fitness moves so that I get an hour into just 30 minutes by combining upper body, lower body, and abdominals simultaneously. I also run and do yoga a couple of times a week, and take one day off for rest and recovery.

My mantra is two part: "I work out because I can" and "Fitness—fit it in!" I can always find ten minutes to sweat or tone, and this keeps me healthy and feeling great!

"I can always find ten minutes to sweat or tone"

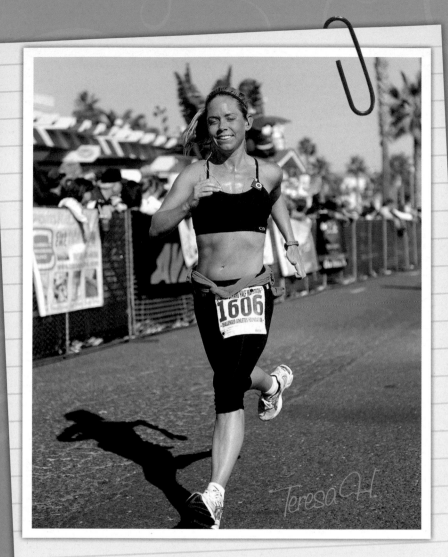

AGE: 33

HEIGHT: 5'4"

WEIGHT: 113 lbs

DRESS SIZE: 0

PROFESSION: nutritional consultant

Teresa H.

I love food! But if I weren't careful about my choices, I'd be gigantic! I studied nutrition in college, as I was most interested in gaining knowledge of how to fuel a healthy body. Ten years after graduation, I found myself 20 pounds overweight. The weight gain can't be attributed to any one thing in particular, other than life. But to take it off, I had to put my skills to work and instill structure into my daily routines. As a result, I lost the 20 pounds in roughly 20 weeks.

Today I eat six times a day: three meals and three snacks. I'm a calorie counter, so I keep my meals between 250 and 400 calories and snacks around 100 to 200. I make sure to get at least 60 grams of protein and 30 grams of fiber, five servings of fruits and veggies, and three dairy servings a day. I even developed a strategy to keep the alcoholic calories to a minimum during social events. I figure if you're going to have a drink or two, why not have half the calories? I also supplement with a multivitamin.

I exercise an hour a day, six days a week. I enjoy running, yoga, spin class, weight lifting, rowing, and the elliptical machine.

I think about my weight often, stepping on the scale first thing in the morning. If the number tips in the wrong direction, I keep a food journal to hold myself accountable, amp up my activity a bit, and aim to not exceed 1400 calories per day until I'm back on track.

"I keep a food journal to hold myself accountable"

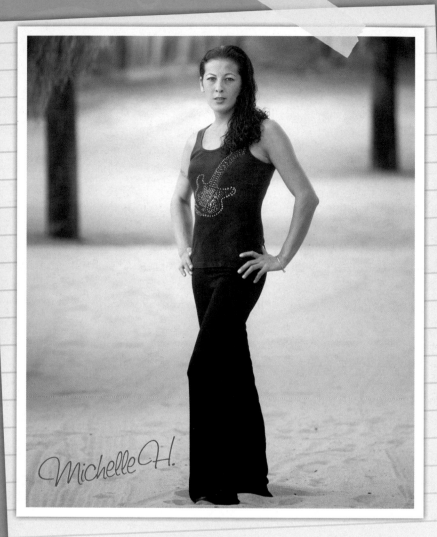

Michelle H.

AGE:	33
HEIGHT:	5'6"
WEIGHT:	120 lbs
DRESS SIZE:	7
# OF CHILDREN:	3
PROFESSION:	home schooling mom, software developer

Michelle H.

Born on the Big Island, I ate fresh vegetables from our garden, seafood, fish, poultry, eggs, brown rice, wheat bread, granola, and fruit. I drank milk, water, and 100% juice, and very rarely had any processed sugar. I learned that the secret to staying healthy was also the key to maintaining a slim and slender body!

To this day, proper nutritional intake is important to me, so I prefer wheat bread, brown and wild rice to anything white, bleached or processed. I prepare a weekly menu in advance to ensure that each food group is consumed daily. I pre-cut vegetables, meats, and snacks such as a variety of sandwiches and peeled carrots and avoid MSG, which is found in junk and fast foods, as it causes me to eat more, and more often. I learned that polluting my body with empty calories leaves me unsatisfied and hungry.

Being active also helps my body's natural process to run smoothly. I realize how much time I spend at my desk, so I replaced my computer chair with an exercise ball and bounce when I browse or spring up and down while watching TV. The results are phenomenal with the ease of feeling like I'm not even exercising at all!

A healthy lifestyle takes focus and effort, but it's important for me to make time for such things. And as a result, I have energy throughout the day to feel—to coin my own special word—phentabulous!

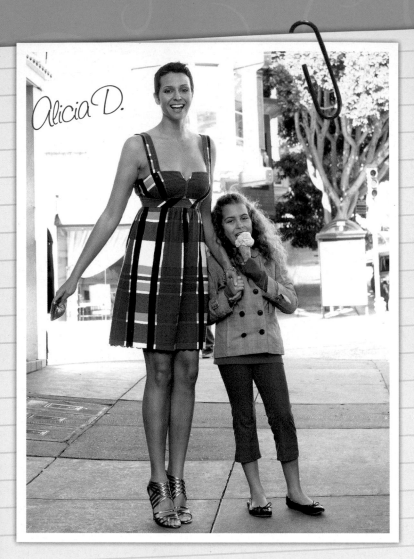

Alicia D.

AGE: 33

HEIGHT: 5'9"

WEIGHT: 135 lbs

DRESS SIZE: 4/6

OF CHILDREN: 1

PROFESSION: author, business coach, self-publishing consultant

Alicia D.

When I was 18, I traveled to Italy to model—and what began as a promising experience soon turned discouraging. Upon arrival, I didn't need an interpreter to figure out that I was too big for their standards, so they sent me home. Frustrated and daunted, I ate even more than usual! But I soon learned that consuming food out of boredom or disappointment only made things worse. So I decided to watch what I ate in conjunction with a solid exercise commitment to keep me feeling and looking my best.

Today I eat most of the foods I want by using the moderation rule. However, I do avoid carbs and dairy, choosing healthier fruits, vegetables, and protein instead. I favor Indian and Mediterranean cuisine and enjoy a good glass of wine. And when I eat out, I make healthy choices such as avoiding the bread, ordering broiled and lightly sautéed over fried foods, and sharing dessert rather than having a whole one on my own.

Although I have thin arms and legs, I'm an apple shape with a tendency for weight to settle around my waistline. Being physically active helps me to counter that, so I am committed to running two to five times a week. I also love yoga and Pilates.

While heredity will always come into play, I use exercise and diet to control my weight, size, and health. It's good for me and is a good example for my daughter.

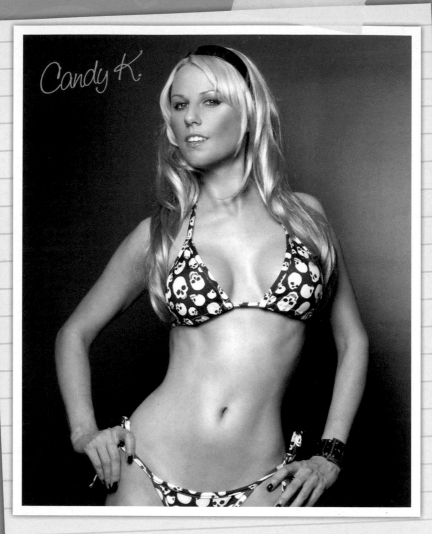

Candy K.

AGE:	34
HEIGHT:	5'9"
WEIGHT:	130 lbs
DRESS SIZE:	4
PROFESSION:	costume designer, clothing line owner

Candy K.

I took thinness for granted until I turned 30, when to my dismay I noticed weight started creeping on. Because I never had to work at it, I had no idea how to make it stop! So I turned to fitness magazines like *Shape* and *Self*, which helped me learn about making better food choices and how to develop a workout plan.

Today I make a concerted effort to avoid sugar and sodium because they make my midsection bloated and cover up the hard work I do to flatten it out. I read food labels when shopping and avoid items containing anything chemical or processed. I enjoy carbs, but substitute whole grains and unbleached flour for a healthier version of my favorites.

I work out first thing in the morning so I don't wimp out after I get home. I warm up with a 15-minute walk followed by 30 to 60 minutes on the Wii Fit, stationary bike, or home rowing machine. I also use a balance ball for my abdominals, and end with 15 minutes of yoga and stretching.

My daily challenge is to keep my body firm. I do this with consistent exercise, and the overall effect keeps me feeling confident and sexy!

"My daily challenge is to keep my body firm."

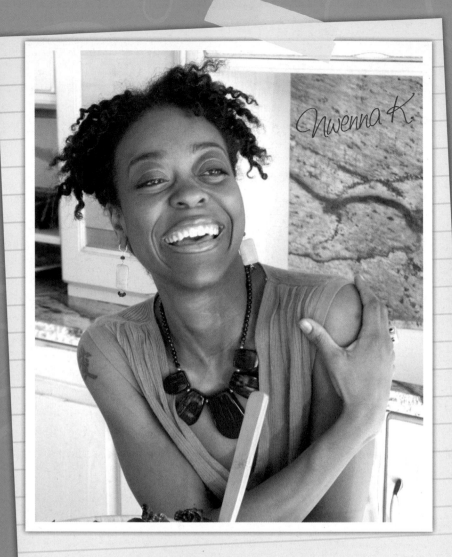

Nwenna K.

AGE: 34
HEIGHT: 5'5"
WEIGHT: 112 lbs
DRESS SIZE: 0/2
PROFESSION: urban eco-culinary activist

Nwenna K.

Growing up, African-American boys of my age desired thicker, fuller girls and I wasn't that type of girl at all! But I couldn't bring myself to eat anything unhealthy or fattening, as it never made me feel very good afterwards. I eventually gravitated toward a vegetarian lifestyle, because that is how I felt the most vibrant and energetic.

Today I eat a mostly raw food diet. I stick to six to eight small meals a day. My favorite foods are beets, seaweed vegetables, avocados, kale, and blueberries. I love fresh food and big salads, and when it comes to veggies, I favor dark leafy greens. When I get cravings, I substitute healthy snacks in place of sweets or salty foods. I drink a lot of water and I take multivitamin powders in my smoothies. I also supplement with liquid kelp, which helps re-establish thyroid balance, which in turn, aids weight loss. It is also excellent for restoring nutrients for healthy hair, nails, and skin.

For exercise I take brisk morning walks, hike, and do Bikram yoga to keep my bones warm. I exercise not only to keep my weight under control, but also because it simply makes me feel so good!

I believe that a health-conscious diet along with regular exercise and a positive outlook on life are the key factors to maintaining my weight.

"Today I eat a mostly raw food diet."

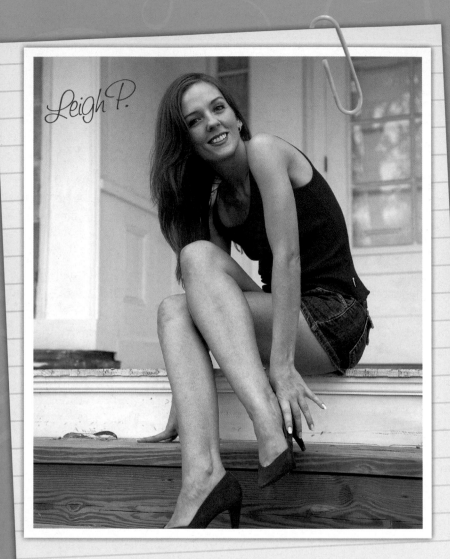

Leigh P.

AGE: 34

HEIGHT: 5'4"

WEIGHT: 105 lbs

DRESS SIZE: 3

PROFESSION: internet marketing expert, vocalist, owner of an online boutique

Leigh P.

Growing up my legs were like toothpicks all the way up to my ribs, so I was encouraged to eat anything at any time. It wasn't until reaching my 30's that I began taking diet and exercise seriously for the sake of long-term well-being.

Today I eat five to six small, healthy meals each day. I drink plenty of water, and make sure to get enough sleep. Breakfast is cereal and toast. I snack on raw veggies or crackers and cheese throughout the day, and for dinner I enjoy some protein-enriched pasta or a healthy sandwich.

I spend a lot of time dancing because that gives me a lot of pleasure, and sometimes do yoga for a balance and a toned core. Posture is important to me, and yoga helps that.

Exercising in a way that I enjoy, getting adequate rest, reading, writing, relaxing, listening to music, and spending time with animals lead me to live a balanced, stress-free life. I love what I do and as long as I maintain my health, I feel great!

"I spend a lot of time dancing."

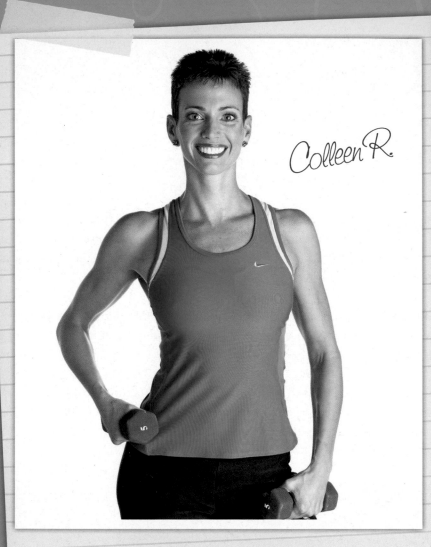

Colleen R.

AGE:	35
HEIGHT:	5'7"
WEIGHT:	124 lbs
DRESS SIZE:	4
PROFESSION:	personal trainer, creator of DVD fitness series for moms

Colleen R.

As a competitive swimmer throughout high school and college, I learned how good it felt to set goals, work hard, and achieve them. And to this day I am an avid exercise enthusiast!

I eat every two and a half to three hours, which keeps my metabolism revving and my blood sugar steady. And in this way I never get to the "Oh my gosh, I must eat a cheeseburger!" feeling. Breakfast is egg whites and oatmeal with cinnamon and blueberries followed by an apple with all natural peanut butter for a snack. Lunch is a piece of Eizekel bread topped with lean protein, tomato, avocado, and a piece of provolone with a spinach salad with pear and strawberries topped with a bit of balsamic vinegar. Another snack is a Kashi bar or nonfat yogurt with cinnamon and fresh fruit. Dinner includes chicken or fish, brown rice, quinoa or a sweet potato, and veggie such as steamed broccoli with fresh squeezed lemon. I stay away from processed foods, white flour, or added sugar. I drink 10–15 cups of water a day; however, I do enjoy my wine on the weekends! As far as supplements, I use Prograde's VGF 25+ multivitamin for Women, Krill Oil, and a post-workout replacement drink. I also love the Life Shotz product from 21TEN for clean, sustained all-day energy.

I lift weights and do cardio, but my favorite and most effective workout is full-body circuit training. I keep the intensity high with lots of heart-pumping moves that include multiple body parts. I also incorporate body-weight exercises like pull-ups, chin-ups, push-ups, and lunges. As far as effective cardio, I find that interval training is best. I warm up for five minutes then do 20 minutes, alternating 30 seconds for sprints, and 30 seconds to recover. It's tough, but it's over quickly!

I don't like to step on a scale, so instead I gauge my weight by the way my clothes fit ,and my health by how I feel. Making a daily action commitment to exercise allows me to maintain the best me I can be!

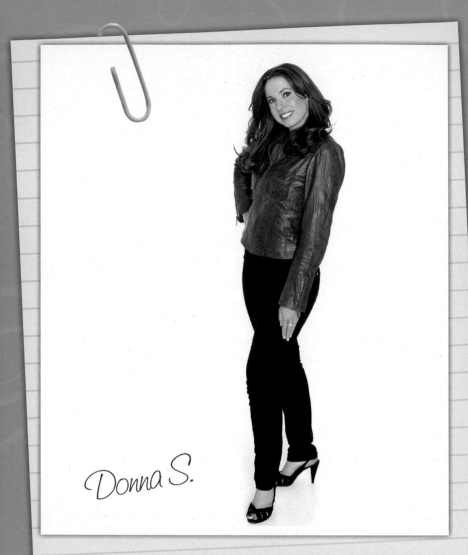

Donna S.

AGE:	36
HEIGHT:	5'5"
WEIGHT:	130 lbs
DRESS SIZE:	6
PROFESSION:	actress, book publishing specialist

Donna S.

I love food! But I make it a point to eat for both taste *and* nutrition. I keep it fresh, organic, homemade, and real by avoiding foods that come out of a can, box, or carton. Often when I cook, I freeze the leftovers in meal-size portions so all I have to do is heat, and voila! When I eat sugar and processed foods I feel sluggish, but when I eat healthily I feel vibrant, my mood improves, and I don't get sick. So proper nutrition is my first and best line of defense.

I live by the beach and after a sand walk or a walk n' talk with a friend, I feel energized. Sometimes I have to drag myself outside, but once I'm there, I'm so glad I did! I also incorporate weights, and that gives me a long, lean and toned look, and I love the results.

For me, it's all about loving my body and giving it what it needs for optimal health. Sure it means giving up Twinkies, but big whoop! After feeling so good and alive when my body is healthy and well nourished, it's just worth the effort.

"Sure it means giving up twinkies, but big whoop!"

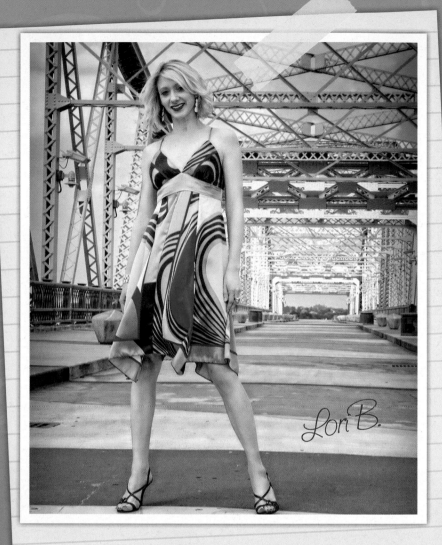

Lori B.

AGE: 36

HEIGHT: 5'3"

WEIGHT: 100 lbs

DRESS SIZE: 2

PROFESSION: image consultant,
career coach

Lori B.

As I was a very picky eater, "Bird Legs," "Knotsy Knees," and "Toothpick" were just a few of the nicknames I had growing up. However, once I got to high school I was determined to fill out. So I convinced my dad to by me some weights and started drinking weight-gaining milkshakes, but it didn't work. When I got to college, I was no longer picky and ate everything, but still could not gain weight! Dinner consisted of one or two entrees, a couple of sides, grilled cheese, and a dessert or two. Before long, I realized I had to incorporate a healthy dose of exercise in order to look not only healthy, but also well proportioned and toned.

Today I no longer eat everything in sight. Rather, I enjoy whole foods and pay attention to stopping when comfortably full. In addition, I drink mostly water and avoid soda. And when I crave sweets, I substitute a healthy alternative such as a tablespoon of Nutella instead of cookies or cake.

When it comes to exercise, I am sporadic. I'll go for a while with a regular routine of working out and then quit it all together for an extended period of time. I've always enjoyed weight training over cardio workouts and can build muscle fast. This past year, however, my workout routine has consisted only of hiking. It's my love of nature and wildlife that keep this form of exercise from getting boring, and I plan to stick with it.

My weight is important to me, it's true, but it's not nearly as vital as my emotional and spiritual health and living a life that is full of joy! See, in the past I felt awkward, scrawny, and unattractive being thin until I finally embraced it. As a skinny person always made fun of, I have learned to develop a healthy body image and not worry about what others say.

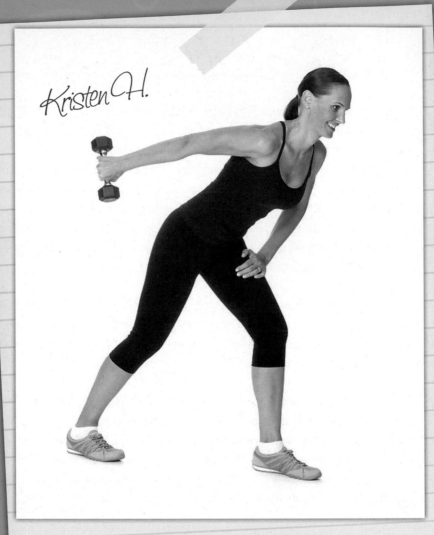

Kristen H.

AGE: 36

HEIGHT: 5'8"

WEIGHT: 140 lbs

DRESS SIZE: 6

OF CHILDREN: 2

PROFESSION: CEO of Baby Boot Camp

Kristen H.

D o you really want to know how often I eat? Nearly every waking hour—seriously! I'm a grazer, and I love food. In fact, after graduating college, I enrolled in a culinary academy and went on to become a pastry chef!

To counteract my ravenous appetite, I drink a lot of liquids. At any given point in time, you will find three or four beverages on my desk such as Pellegrino, a 24-oz stainless steel water bottle, or my favorite—green tea powder with lemon and agave nectar. I avoid wheat and gluten, and supplement with Omega-3 fish oil.

My exercise routine includes KARNA CAMP (a small group training for women), Baby Boot Camp (a stroller-based fitness for mom and baby), spin class, and interval training. I also jog, using a run/walk method to prevent injury.

I not only exercise to maintain my weight, but also my health. In addition, being physically active helps aid my digestion. Setting short-term fitness goals causes me to think about food as fuel, and sleep as recovery. As a result, I take better care of my body, and the outcome is that I am a happier and more energetic me!

"Being physically active helps aid my digestion"

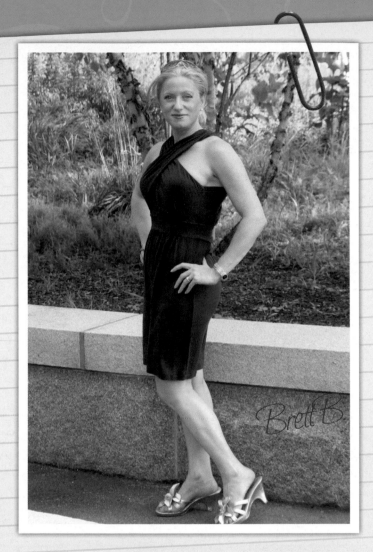

AGE: 36

HEIGHT: 5'3"

WEIGHT: 125 lbs

DRESS SIZE: 4

PROFESSION: health and wellness expert

Brett B.

I wasn't overweight growing up, but I wasn't a skinny-mini either. When I got to college, I became aware of healthy eating and exercise for the purpose of releasing stress and doing well in school. As a result, I started paying attention to what I ate, and fell in love with health and wellness.

Today I am a mastermind at reading nutrition labels, and stick to whole foods while minimizing refined sugars and anything processed. I maintain my weight by following these guidelines:

- I eat four to six small meals a day, ensuring that each contains some healthy fat such as Omega-3s or monounsaturated fats, lean protein, and fiber.
- I get at least 25 grams of fiber a day, mostly from vegetables and whole fruit.
- I eat a lot of vegetables, but limit those that are starchy such as potatoes and corn. I go for grains in their least processed form such as whole oats, flaxseed, and brown rice. I also enjoy fruits rich in antioxidants (such as berries) and love nuts, olives, and beans.
- I maintain a diet balanced in this way: 40–60% carbohydrates, 30–40% protein, and 20–30% fat.
- I exercise 45 minutes to an hour, five to six times a week, incorporating strength training on at least three of those days. As well, I aim to sleep for a minimum of seven to eight hours per night.

I look at my life as a whole, so my long-term wellness strategy includes a holistic approach that addresses both body and mind. And although I maintain healthy eating habits, I allow myself to indulge 15% of the time, which gives me the freedom to enjoy life without feeling deprived!

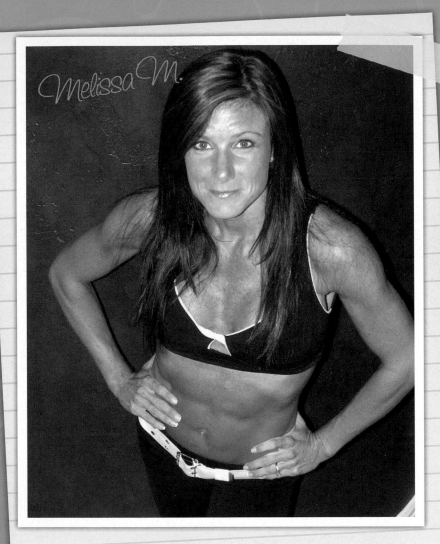

Melissa M.

AGE:	36
HEIGHT:	5'7"
WEIGHT:	140 lbs
DRESS SIZE:	4
# OF CHILDREN:	2
PROFESSION:	health, fitness, and life coach

Melissa M.

rowing up, I avoided physical exertion. I didn't like to sweat! It wasn't until I had children that I decided on exercise to get that baby weight off. It took trial and error to find something I enjoyed doing, but once I did, nothing could keep me away from it! I also changed my eating habits. At first I didn't like the taste of less-processed foods, so I committed to eating cleaner for 30 days, just to hold myself accountable. I was pleasantly surprised to find I had more energy and felt so much better at the end of the month!

Today I am a big fan of protein and eating five times each day. Each meal comes from lean protein, veggies, fruit, and whole grains. I have Shakeology (a meal replacement shake) after every workout and never eat past 8 p.m. And as I'm on the run, I find, dauntingly, that fructose corn syrup and trans-fat are in most every convenience food. So I make a commitment to be mindful by preparing healthy snacks and bringing them with me. I also drink more water than Shamu the whale!

Since finding a program I enjoy, exercising has become fun for me! My favorite class is Turbo Kick kickboxing where I bust out a few punches every day to release stress and built-up energy. This is key to helping me keep off those pounds I shed, and has allowed me to stay lean ever since.

Getting back to simpler eating and finding enjoyable activities that make me sweat are the main components to my long-term health plan. After all, I'd rather be taking stairs two at a time than popping pills!

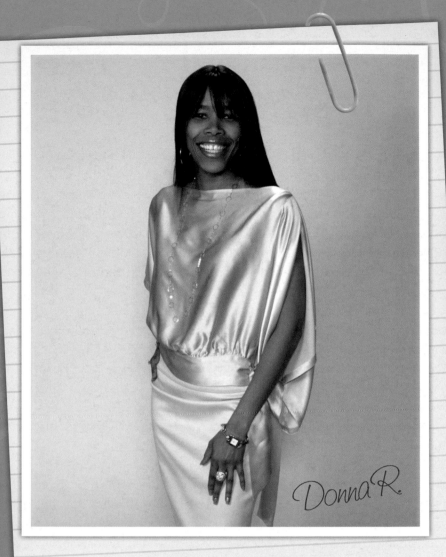

Donna R.

AGE:	37
HEIGHT:	5'6"
WEIGHT:	123 lbs
DRESS SIZE:	0
# OF CHILDREN:	1
PROFESSION:	corporate leadership and team development specialist

Donna R.

I have been slim most of my life, except for three times: freshman year of college, my first year in the army, and when I was pregnant. To lose the weight each time, I did three things: exercised, changed my eating habits, and gave away the fat clothes!

Today I eat three meals and three snacks a day. For breakfast I have oatmeal and herbal tea, followed by a mid-morning snack of either a banana or an apple with peanut butter. Lunch is baked chicken, potatoes, and a vegetable followed by a handful of raw carrots or nuts mid- afternoon. Dinner is lean protein either baked or sautéed with olive oil, and I finish the night with fruit. I do not count calories but minimize the amount of sugar and boxed food that I consume. I also drink eight glasses of water daily and rarely drink alcohol.

I exercise three to four times a week, which includes weight training, cardio, and calisthenics. I do abdominal work to keep the stomach flat and squats to firm the derrière. I do not own a scale and only weigh myself at annual check-ups.

It may sound funny, but I try on my prom dress every three months to make sure that it still fits. This has been one of my motivating factors to staying thin!

"Today I eat three meals and three snacks a day."

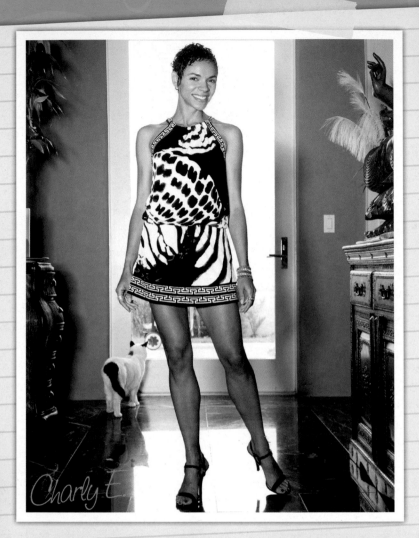

Charly E.

AGE:	38
HEIGHT:	5'2"
WEIGHT:	98 lbs
DRESS SIZE:	2
PROFESSION:	personal strategist, TV personality

Charly E.

I took dance classes as a kid and was always quite thin. However, my weight battle started the moment I hit puberty when my hips and thighs started filling out. By the time I reached my mid-twenties, I'd packed an extra 45 pounds onto my petite frame! I was a yo-yo dieting pro until one day I saw an older woman in a tennis outfit—looking most fit and fabulous. That was the day I called Jenny Craig. It took just under six months to lose the weight, but the real achievement has been keeping it off.

Today I eat small meals at least five times a day to boost my metabolism. My diet consists of poultry, fish, fruits, and vegetables such as broccoli, spinach, cabbage, and squash. I love crunchy, simple carbs, so I add rice crackers and spelt toast to my meals. I cook with either olive or coconut oil, and minimize foods with fake contents created in labs. So if it's going to be butter, it's the real thing! Getting used to smaller portions prevents me from overeating when I eat out. Doggie bag please! I supplement with a multivitamin, chlorella, fish oil, and DHEA.

I commit to four days a week of either Pilates, a spin class, or brisk walks. A variety of activity keeps me exercising regularly without burning out.

I feel best when my focus shifts from the scale to treating myself well. Therefore I make a mental check before choosing what foods to consume. And when my weight goes up, I eat smaller portions and increase my exercise until I comfortably fit back into my clothes again. Awareness and accountability have allowed me to experience long-term weight loss without exercise or food dominating my thoughts—or my life.

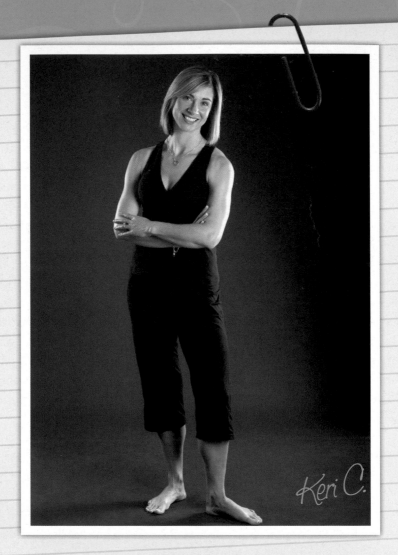

AGE: 38

HEIGHT: 5'9"

WEIGHT: 135 lbs

OF CHILDREN: 1

PROFESSION: fitness instructor

Keri C.

I enjoyed being physically active growing up, and to this day I'm still a fitness enthusiast!

I eat three meals and two snacks each day. I consider myself to be a fairly healthy eater—not a lot of red meat, not a lot of fast food. My snacks are usually in the form of a bar, which equals quick energy, no mess, and can be eaten in the car. I don't eat soy, but will eat an occasional yogurt. When eating out I order meals without sauce, mayonnaise, or condiments, and ask for dressing on the side. When indulging in carbs, I make certain they are of the complex variety such as whole wheat over white. I drink water all day, and take a daily multivitamin along with glucosamine and chondroitin to aid with joint stiffness.

I run, hike, spin, core train, and do Pilates and/or aerobics five days a week.

I weigh myself once a week on the same scale where I work, and ultimately judge my weight daily by how my jeans fit. I have always been thin, but it is dedication to exercise that makes me look fit. I work very hard for my curves!

"...ultimately judge my weight daily by how my jeans fit."

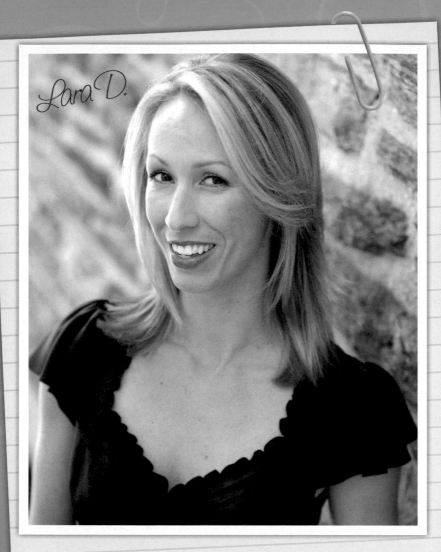

Lara D.

AGE:	38
HEIGHT:	5'9"
WEIGHT:	144 lbs
DRESS SIZE:	6/8
PROFESSION:	owner of a holistic health counseling and fitness practice for busy people

Lara D.

I never struggled with my weight growing up. Once off to college, I did gain that freshman 15, but my weight has remained relatively stable since then. In my early 30's, I made a conscious choice to eat cleanly and healthily. Today I shop mostly organic and natural at places such as Whole Foods and farmer's markets. I have settled on a few simple rules that help me maintain a well-balanced approach to my weight:

- I eat whatever I like—in moderation.
- I listen to my body; it tells me what works for me and what doesn't.
- I eat high-quality carbohydrates like whole grains, fruits, and veggies.
- I eat mostly plant proteins, adding fish, lean meat, and dairy products a couple times a week.
- I eat fresh, organic foods whenever possible, avoiding anything processed.
- I eat slowly and savor my food.

For breakfast, I have a bowl of oatmeal with fresh fruit and nuts. For lunch, I have a veggie burger or turkey sandwich, sushi, or a bean-based vegetarian dish. A mid-afternoon snack is either fruit or a handful of nuts. And for dinner, I have fish, beans, or tofu, plus a grain and veggie. I keep portion sizes reasonable, and drink water, never soda (but I do drink coffee in the morning!). I don't count calories, but I read labels like a hawk, which helps me avoid overly processed foods. I steer clear of sugar in favor of sweeteners like brown rice syrup, agave nectar, and honey, and take a multivitamin and calcium to supplement.

I walk to get from place to place, do Pilates, and run three to four miles a few times a week. If I start to notice my weight creeping up, I just pay a little more attention to what I eat and how much.

My bottom line is balance. Taking care of myself just makes me feel better, both physically and mentally. And that's all the motivation I need to stick with a healthy diet and consistent exercise!

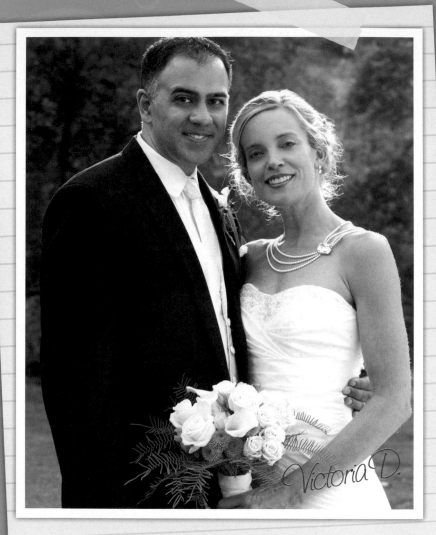

Victoria D.

AGE:	39
HEIGHT:	5'4"
WEIGHT:	118 lbs
DRESS SIZE:	2/4
PROFESSION:	physician

Victoria D.

Although I was of average size growing up, by my early thirties my weight began redistributing and settling around my middle. Even when I exercised regularly, I couldn't get rid of my "spare tire." Because I was working crazy hours, I'd skip breakfast and seldom eat lunch. As a result, I would feel shaky and lightheaded, and by the time I got home I'd be so hungry that I'd eat a big dinner and continue to snack until bedtime. Skipping meals, lack of sleep, stress, and eating the wrong carbs were enough to cause harm. As a physician, I knew it boiled down to erratic insulin and blood sugar levels that lead to carbohydrate cravings, but it was quite by accident that I started losing weight from some supplements I started. I soon became well-schooled in the relationship between metabolism, blood sugar, and weight control.

Within the first week of taking a pharmaceutical grade multivitamin/mineral/antioxidant blend, I not only lost weight, but slowly regained my energy levels as well. I no longer crashed at work and I ate less at night. I began reading more about the ingredients in the blend that helped maintain stable blood sugar—chromium, magnesium, vitamin D, resveratrol, grape seed extract, and other phytonutrients. This knowledge convinced me to try some related weight-management meal replacements, namely high fiber/high protein shakes. The combination kept my blood sugar stable all day long, and then the weight *really* started to come off! Today, I am at my slimmest since junior high school.

The essential rules I now follow are:

- I eat every two to three hours, five times a day (usually with one or two meal-replacement shakes per day).
- I start the day with a low-glycemic meal (lean protein and/or healthy fats, or a shake) to prevent either a spike or a drop in blood sugar.
- The more fiber I ingest, the better for blood sugar control. Multiple doses work better than one big dose.
- I take a complete vitamin/mineral blend, divided twice daily.
- I minimize refined carbohydrates and processed foods.
- I don't keep any junk food in the house.
- Feeling hungry means I have waited too long to eat, so I adjust my schedule accordingly.

For exercise I walk a few times a week, but that's it. For me, meal-replacement shakes work because I don't have time to consistently prepare healthy, balanced meals. If I start craving everything in sight (like over the holidays), I remind myself how addicting sugar can be. Then I get super-strict for a couple of days, and the cravings disappear again.

For me, the key to staying slim is managing the cravings, which can only happen if my blood sugar is stable. I was on a mission to tackle this problem, and was successful. Now I'm excited to share with others how to manage weight successfully—without feeling tortured!

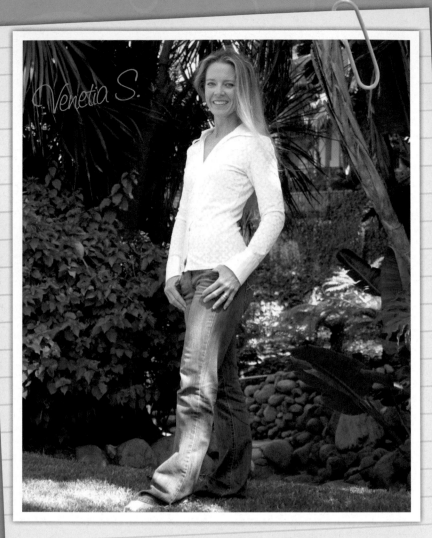

Venetia S.

AGE: 39
HEIGHT: 5'3"
WEIGHT: 113 lbs
DRESS SIZE: 4/6
OF CHILDREN: 2
PROFESSION: domestic engineer

Venetia S.

Growing up, I was happily involved with numerous sports activities. However, after becoming a mom, I gained some unwanted weight. I found that 30 minutes of exercise a few times a week was a must, so I sought out a pool and did laps. I also got an infant jogger and a bicycle with a baby trailer so I would have no excuses. The plan worked wonders!

Today I have five to six small meals a day. Breakfast is organic steel-cut oats with fruit. For a mid-morning snack, I have a whey protein shake and a handful of raw almonds. For lunch I incorporate protein, fat, and a small amount of carbs, such as an egg salad sandwich, followed by yogurt late afternoon. For dinner I have grilled chicken with couscous and a green vegetable. I cut bread out of my diet, substituting a few small crackers or tortillas instead. I also eliminated sugar, using honey, applesauce, and stevia as a substitute. I avoid drinking anything that includes artificial colors, flavorings or fructose. I drink a lot of water instead, flavoring it with fresh lemon or a splash of caffeine-free tea. I supplement with Omega 3-6-9, and vitamins B and C.

I allocate an hour a day for exercise by either taking morning walks or going to the gym. Once there, I do 10 minutes on the treadmill, then alternate five-minute run/walks back and forth for about 30 minutes. I like variety so I switch it up with weight training and swimming for 30 minutes four to five times a week.

I don't think about my weight every day, but don't ignore it either. I enjoy the mental clarity that comes with physical exertion, and think about the good I'm doing for my body. And when I'm tempted by treats, I may indulge a bit, as I like to enjoy life! But every day I consciously work at keeping myself in the best condition I can be.

"Movement is a medicine for creating change in a person's physical, emotional, and mental states."

~ Carol Welch

The 40's

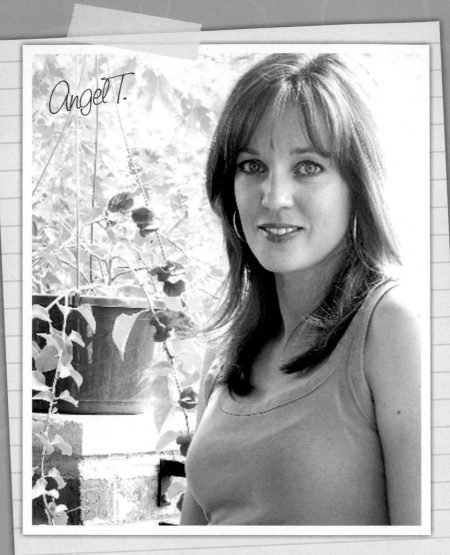

Angel T.

AGE: 40

HEIGHT: 5'1"

WEIGHT: 107 lbs

DRESS SIZE: 4

OF CHILDREN: 3

PROFESSION: radio show host, author

Angel T.

I have always been thin, but watched my maternal lineage get thicker and thicker with age. So, using my family heredity as my virtual mirror, I set out to change my legacy. Each day I ate smaller, healthier portions than before, rarely finished everything on my plate, and made a special point to stop when I felt full. Eventually these strategies became habit-forming and today I can say that I'm proud of my health, energy and figure.

For breakfast I have a scrambled egg or half a whole-wheat English muffin with peanut butter and apple slices. For lunch I have a salad with a variety of veggies. I use dressing sparingly and skip the cheese. I drink a lot of water all day and enjoy hot tea with lemon when the weather gets cold. I avoid soda but do enjoy the occasional glass of wine.

Jogging is the perfect exercise for me, so each week I schedule a three-mile run. The other days I add in activities such as tennis, yoga, walking, or the elliptical machine. I'm able to maintain my physique as long as I'm active for at least 30 minutes a day.

I don't own a scale, but my clothes tell me when it's time to increase my activity or watch what I'm eating. When my pants get tight, my motto is to eat less and exercise more!

"Eventually these strategies became habit-forming."

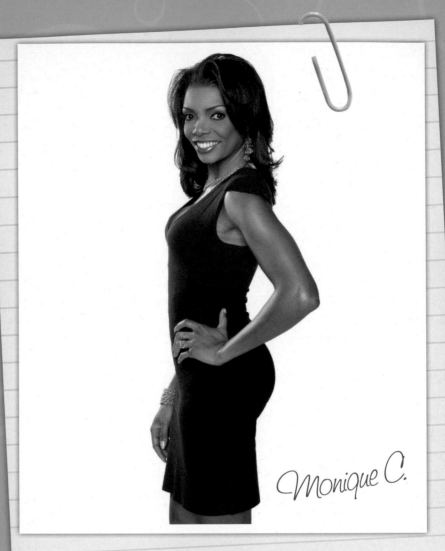

Monique C.

AGE:	40
HEIGHT:	5'6"
WEIGHT:	130 lbs
DRESS SIZE:	4
# OF CHILDREN:	1
PROFESSION:	producer, media coach, TV and radio personality

Monique C.

I grew up indulging in all varieties of soul food such as burgers, pizza, fried pork chops, and my favorites—Chicago-style hot dogs and Maxwell Street polish sausages— yummy! I never had a reason to worry about my weight, or so I thought! When I got to college I developed a bit of a pouch. A visit to the doctor proved I had gained almost 30 lbs—I was going down the wrong road! I decided to take action because I felt miserable and didn't want to be overweight and unhealthy. So I stopped drinking soda and opted for salads over burgers and raw or steamed veggies over the ones cooked so long they lost their color. I also started to appreciate the benefits of water and began drinking a lot of it. I also hired a personal trainer to encourage me and hold me accountable. It took about a year to lose the weight, and in the process I really got the importance of:

- eating four to six small, nutritious meals every day, which helps speed metabolism and keeps the body constantly burning calories.
- drinking a minimum of eight glasses of water per day. When I doubled my water intake, my body flushed itself out and the weight began to melt off.
- weight training instead of just cardio. Yes, the treadmill helps the body lose weight but if that's all one does, muscle will also be lost and the end result is flab. Weight training helps tone, strengthen, and burn fat, even while the body rests.
- staying away from processed food. White flour, rice, sugar, bread should be eliminated from any diet as they do not help maintain health! I avoid these foods and opt for brown rice, wheat bread, and natural sweeteners like maple syrup or agave by Wholesome Sweeteners.
- supplements. The correct nutritionals such as a good multivitamin should be taken daily to support optimal health and vitality. I started taking one and since doing so, I have more energy than I did when I was 25!

I commit to working out for an hour at least three to four days a week. As a result, I have formidable muscle tone, energy, vitality, and an unprecedented zest for life.

I'm excited every day that I can show people how beautiful, strong, and fit a woman can be at 40 and beyond. Yes, my natural thinness is back, but more importantly, I have regained optimal health, and now eating well and staying active is a way of life!

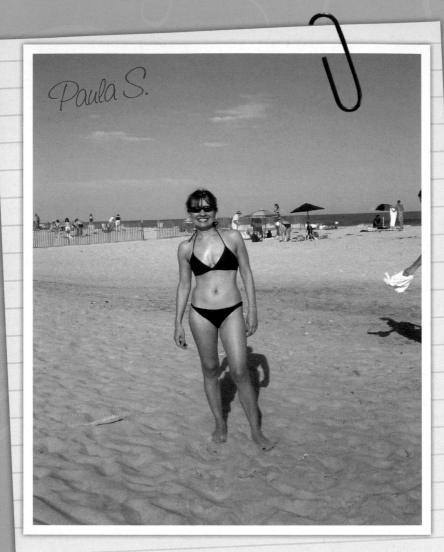

Paula S.

AGE:	40
HEIGHT:	5'3"
WEIGHT:	105 lbs
DRESS SIZE:	2
PROFESSION:	real estate professional

Paula S.

As a kid I was encouraged to eat a lot of fruits and veggies, and portion sizes were served small. Dessert was for treats and special occasions, and to this day, I maintain the same healthy-eating philosophy: Staying away from junk food is key!

Today I continue to treat food seriously. I have a protein drink with either water or coconut milk for breakfast. I snack on nuts and power bars, and always carry them with me, as I never want to feel hungry. I avoid soy, limit dairy, and with that, stick to only fat-free versions. I avoid sugar, and when I do have carbs, I only consume the whole-wheat and brown rice variety. I drink water and green tea during the day, but wouldn't dream of having a soda. I read food labels and avoid all things processed. I don't drink alcohol much—one glass with dinner a couple of times a week is my limit. And I supplement with a daily multivitamin and some antioxidants.

I exercise three to five times a week with boot camp, boxing, or body sculpture classes at the gym, and during the summer I enjoy tennis, hiking, rock climbing, and mountain biking.

I generally have a happy disposition, and have found that a combination of appetite control, attitude, and activity enables me to maintain a healthy state of both mind and body!

"staying away from junk food is key!"

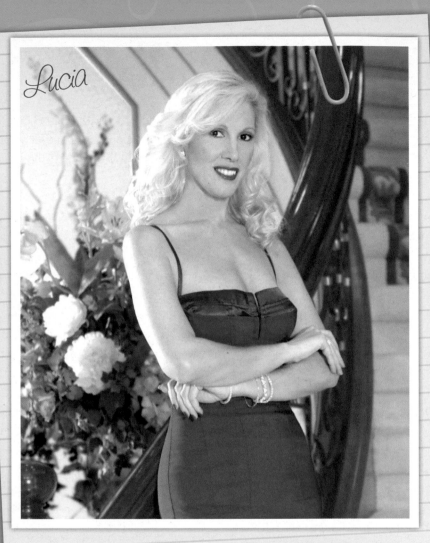

Lucia

AGE:	I don't believe that a woman should reveal her age.
HEIGHT:	5'6"
WEIGHT:	125 lbs
DRESS SIZE:	4
PROFESSION:	dating and relationship expert

Lucia

Growing up I was stick thin. However, when I reached my teens, I became aware of the importance of exercise for good health, so I began jogging. Later I began working out with weights and ended up loving the results. That was enough motivation to make a lifestyle change, and I have kept it up for the last couple of decades.

I graze throughout the day, eating every few hours. I eat a high-protein, low-carb diet consisting of broccoli, egg whites, whole-grain bread, salad, avocados, blueberries, yogurt, Irish oatmeal, steamed vegetables, chicken, and baby carrots. I drink almond milk, water and tea, avoiding soda, fruit juice, and anything containing high-fructose corn syrup. I don't add sugar or salt to anything, and avoid processed or partially-hydrogenated foods like there's no tomorrow! I take supplements such as calcium and antioxidants, and every other month, I throw in a colon or liver cleanse for purification. I'm able to eat cleanly because I don't buy any junk or keep processed foods around. My philosophy: If I don't buy it, then I can't eat it!

I work out a couple of hours a day, and take a dance class twice a week. I also drink plenty of water while exercising.

I've found both a diet and enjoyable exercise that I can stick with and feel comfortable doing long-term. And as long as I get enough rest, I continue to feel good about my body and my health!

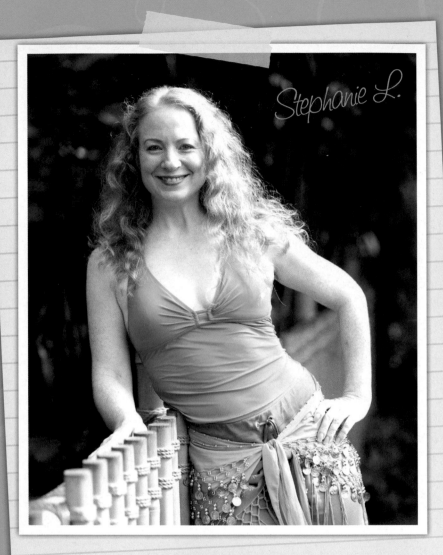

Stephanie L.

AGE: 41
HEIGHT: 5'7"
WEIGHT: 110 lbs
DRESS SIZE: 4
OF CHILDREN: 4
PROFESSION: dancer, prenatal fitness expert

Stephanie L.

As a teen I took ballet and ran track, which kept me slim throughout high school. After I got married, I danced during pregnancy, birth, and postpartum, and gently allowed myself ample time to regain my former physique.

Today I cater to my own appetite and enjoy grazing throughout the day. I eat organic raw fruits and vegetables, seeds, nuts, legumes, beans, and seafood—the more colors and flavors on my plate, the better. I eat something green at every meal (such as a handful of sprouts with breakfast), drink water when thirsty and adore fresh juice. I prepare delectables like sliced beets, julienned dark greens with olive oil, quinoa, tabouleh salad, lentils, and radishes with lime juice and sea salt, so they'll be ready when I get a hunger pang. I don't worry about portion control; however, I do not keep soda in the house, consume caffeine, smoke, drink alcohol, or buy prepared or processed foods.

I dance several times a week for exercise, but more importantly, I do it because I love it! In addition to dancing, I also enjoy walking and yoga. Plus, staying on the move just gives me more energy!

To sum it all up, lots of fruits, veggies, and dancing are delights that require no will power for me. I listen to my intuitive knowledge of what gives me joy and I honor that!

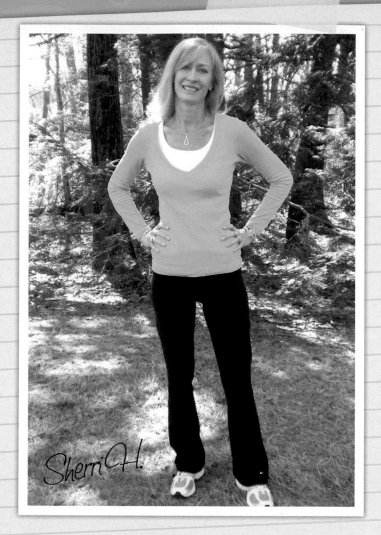

Sherri H.

AGE:	42
HEIGHT:	5'9"
WEIGHT:	125 lbs
DRESS SIZE:	4
# OF CHILDREN:	2
PROFESSION:	mom, blogger, Web site owner

Sherri H.

I was always skinny to the point of being shapeless, so in college I took up anaerobic exercise to build muscle in order to be healthy and not just thin, and that was when fitness became a priority to me.

Today I eat at regular intervals to keep my metabolism going. A typical breakfast is a bowl of whole-grain cereal and a cup of coffee. For lunch, I have all-natural peanut butter on whole wheat bread or a salad with protein. I snack on whole-wheat crackers, carrots, yogurt, fruit, and nuts. For dinner, I choose veggies and lean meats such as chicken or turkey. I avoid processed foods and those that include trans-fats or high-fructose corn syrup. During the day I stick to drinking water, but do enjoy a red wine on occasion. I also take a multivitamin and an omega-3 supplement.

I love the way exercising and working out with weights makes me feel. And if I start to slack off and feel like I'm looking soft and unconditioned, I get back into gear quick! For me, it's not about the weight. Rather, if I feel and look fit, I feel confident and happy with myself.

Maintaining a healthy lifestyle is important to me, not only so that I can feel good, but also so I can set a good example for my children!

"I can set a good example for my children!"

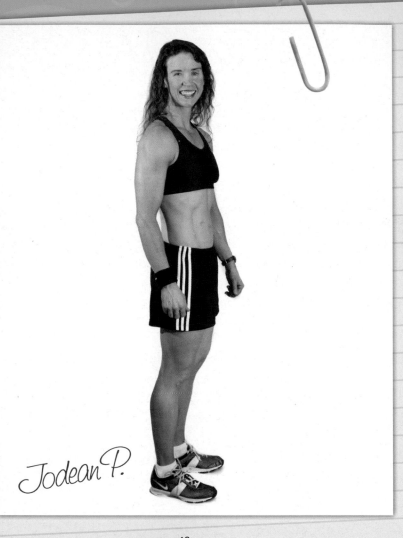

Jodean P.

AGE:	43
HEIGHT:	5'6"
WEIGHT:	125 lbs
DRESS SIZE:	4
PROFESSION:	clinical administrator, author

Jodean P.

When I decided to get fit, I started a food journal. I quickly recognized my inconsistencies and stopped engaging in food activities that were keeping me from my goals. For example, I began politely refusing cake at birthday celebrations and refrained from pasta orders at restaurants.

Today I eat every three hours so as to not get too hungry and avoid cravings. For breakfast I prepare a blueberry, spinach, and whey protein shake. Lunch is a chicken salad and some almonds. For dinner, I have lean protein and a salad of purple cabbage, spinach, green leafy lettuce, onions, bell peppers, tomatoes, and walnuts. I drink at least eight glasses of water a day, plenty of green tea, and never, EVER have soda.

Each morning, I go to the gym and do 30 to 45 minutes of cardio followed by circuit training. I've learned that using more weight and resting less burns more calories, so I follow this regimen and end up nicely toned.

The keys to my slimness are weight-bearing exercises, small portion sizes, keeping sugar intake to a minimum, and making sure I get plenty of rest. I feel strong and healthy and this gives me the motivation I need to keep going. And I'm always flattered when people compliment me on my body and ask me how I do it!

"I began politely refusing cake at birthday celebrations"

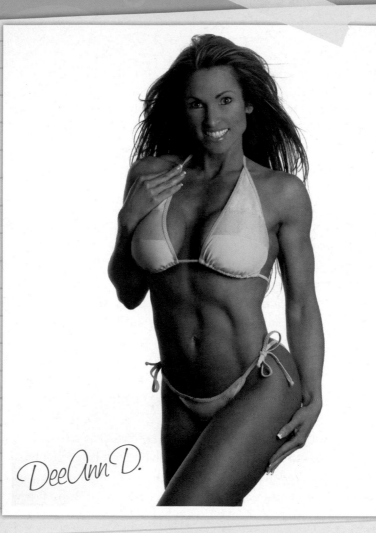

DeeAnn D.

AGE:	43
HEIGHT:	5'3"
WEIGHT:	115 lbs
DRESS SIZE:	2/4
# OF CHILDREN:	3
PROFESSION:	fitness model, personal trainer, life coach, radio and TV personality

DeeAnn D.

I haven't always been in good shape. In fact, it wasn't until after having children that I discovered exercise! After reading *The Secret of the Ages*, I created a dream journal—a sketchbook of photos and phrases of what I wanted to accomplish in life. I also kept a food log where I wrote down everything I ate and all exercises I did. This completely transformed my lifestyle and I have never looked back!

Today I eat six times a day. My diet consists of proteins such as chicken, turkey, egg whites, and whey protein shakes, which allow me to stay lean without water retention. I stick to healthy carbs such as brown rice, oatmeal, apples, and baked potatoes, and I include a salad at both lunch and dinner. I make sure to consume good fats such as olive oil and nuts, and supplement with a daily multivitamin. I also drink at least six glasses of water per day.

For exercise, I hit the treadmill for 40 minutes or high-repetition strength training for about an hour a day. However, I make it a point to constantly change up my routine in an effort to stave off monotony.

I have learned the importance of putting myself first when it comes to daily workouts, healthy nutritional eating, and living my own dreams. When people ask me how I do it, I simply reply that I enjoy teaching my children the importance of living a healthy lifestyle!

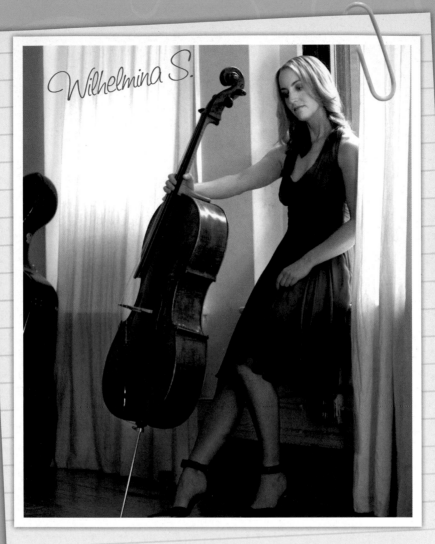

Wilhelmina S.

AGE:	43
HEIGHT:	5'4"
WEIGHT:	110 lbs
DRESS SIZE:	4/6
# OF CHILDREN:	2
PROFESSION:	cellist

Wilhelmina S.

As a young girl, my ballet teacher suggested my mother feed me milkshakes because I was too thin, even by ballerina standards! It wasn't until I had children that I started to notice my metabolism slowing down and some weight creeping in on the problem areas—stomach and posterior! Since then, I have made a concerted effort to stay at my pre-pregnancy weight.

I eat three meals a day and rarely snack. Breakfast is toast or cereal and lunch is soup or salad with baked chips on the side. Dinner is a balance of protein and vegetables and the occasional healthy carb such as whole-wheat pasta with homemade sauce.

I work out a couple of times a week at a gym, as well as take a power walk in the evening. I also do abdominal exercises every day. With me, variety is best, but I do everything in moderation. And if my jeans get snug, I just lower my intake of food and exercise more for a couple of days.

When I look good, I feel good. And when I exercise and work out, I notice that I have fewer physical problems, which is all the motivation I need. And when I do one good thing for my body, it makes me want to do more!

"with me, variety is best, but I do everything in moderation"

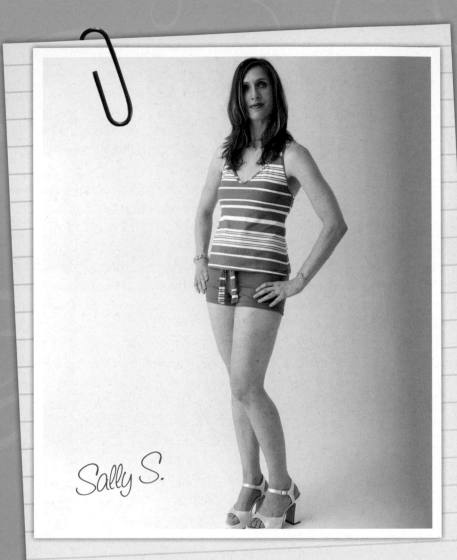

Sally S.

AGE: 43

HEIGHT: 5'3"

WEIGHT: 120 lbs

DRESS SIZE: 6

OF CHILDREN: 2

PROFESSION: jazz pianist, composer, mom, speaker, author, publicity coach, home-biz owner

Sally S.

I did gymnastics as a kid. When I got to college I became a vegetarian, but didn't have a clue what I was doing. I remember eating white rice and butter (YUCK!) and wow, did I gain weight! After graduation I decided to study healthy vegetarianism and learned a lot about nutrition, supplementation, and how whole, uncooked foods can fuel your body and make you feel fantastic. I lost a lot of weight and never felt better! But after getting married and having children, I reverted back to eating the two dreaded Ps: pizza and pasta! I pretty much gained all the weight back until I finally cracked the code to shedding and keeping off those unwanted pounds. Today I've settled on a few basic things that help me maintain my weight. And those things are:

- To keep my body from storing fat cells, I eat every two and a half hours.
- To eliminate cravings, I eat protein bars and drink meal-replacement shakes.
- I avoid anything white such as bread, pasta, sugar, and salt.
- I exercise every other day, alternating between weight-bearing exercises and cardio such as kempo karate or plyometrics (exercising that enables the muscle to reach maximum strength in as short a time as possible).
- I supplement with Life Shotz: a B and D vitamin blend that gives my body the energy it needs to sustain a regular workout schedule, as well as omega-3, calcium, and a good multivitamin.
- I get plenty of sleep—at least eight hours a night.
- And I watch my portion sizes for sure. If I get hungry before bed, I take a tablespoon of protein powder and blend it with some ice and a few frozen berries.

For exercise I like variety, so I have a bunch of Beachbody videos such as Tony Horton's P90X, Shaun T's Hip Hop Abs, Chalene Johnson's Turbo Jam and Debbie Siebers's Slim in 6. And whenever I feel tired or lazy, I think to myself, "Do ya LIKE your new body? Then get off your butt and JUST PUSH PLAY!" And I do.

Yes, staying in shape is hard work, but so worth it!

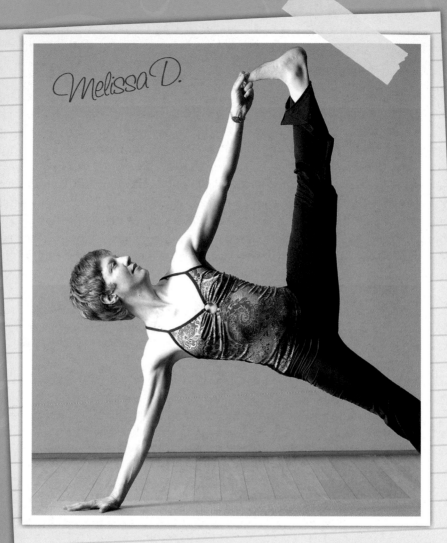

Melissa D.

AGE: 43

HEIGHT: 5'8"

WEIGHT: 130 lbs

DRESS SIZE: 6

PROFESSION: artist, designer, jazz vocalist, freelance writer

Melissa D.

I was always on the thin side. But today it's very important to me to remain fit in addition to being slim, so I exercise regularly and stick to "Paleo" fare, which helps keep my weight consistent. I do allow myself occasional splurges of decadence; however, it's just not all the time!

My diet is mostly vegetarian, although I occasionally eat some fish. I used to avoid oils and fats, but now fat is fair game, so instead I stay away from grains and starchy carbs. I also keep my sugar intake to a minimum and supplement with a multivitamin, calcium, magnesium, omega-7, and estrotone to keep my skin and tissues hydrated.

I take a couple visits to the gym each week for an hour of cardio using the stationary bike, cross- trainer, or stair climber. I also do yoga and walk regularly.

As long as I keep my exercise routines consistent and don't splurge on comfort foods too much, I maintain a healthy, lean figure!

"I stay away from grains and starchy carbs."

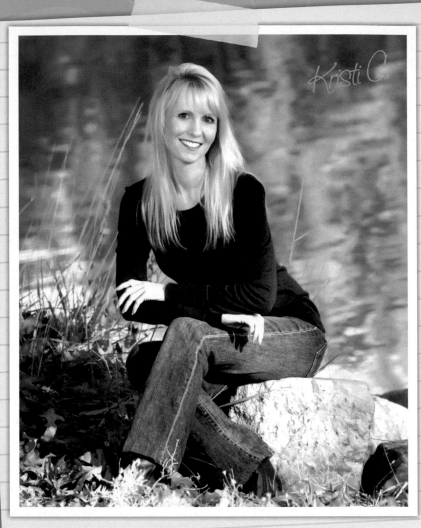

Kristi C

AGE:	43
HEIGHT:	5'4"
WEIGHT:	100 lbs
DRESS SIZE:	0/1
# OF CHILDREN:	5
PROFESSION:	author, speaker, professional certified health coach, single mother of five

Kristi C.

I grew up dancing and remember that constant pressure to stay slim for the next performance. You could have called me a yo-yo dieter at the time! I was active, but never achieved consistency with my weight until I learned a few critical secrets. IgG food allergy testing made a big difference when it came to maintaining my ideal body weight by omitting the foods to which I react unfavorably—like gluten.

Today I maintain a healthy lifestyle by applying a few basic principles. I eat only when I'm hungry and exercise regularly. I stay away from sugar and fats while drinking tons of water—I take a bottle with me wherever I go. Whole foods and supplements are another key for me.

I exercise a minimum of four days a week. Either I jog, go to the gym, or do a home video workout. At the gym, I begin with abdominal work, followed by upper body and legs for about 30 minutes. Then I on move to the treadmill inclined 8 to 25 degrees for 30 minutes. This works the back of the gluts and thighs which produces a great result—a firm, well-defined derriere! At home I use a workout video—rotating between high- and low-impact routines along with a separate abdominal tape every time. My stomach is flatter now working out in this way than before I ever had any of my five children!

I weigh myself often, but focus on how I look more than the scale results. I determine where I want to tone, and then concentrate on those areas. Staying in shape is hard, but well worth the effort, as exercising and eating proper foods afford me the ability to feel good both physically and mentally.

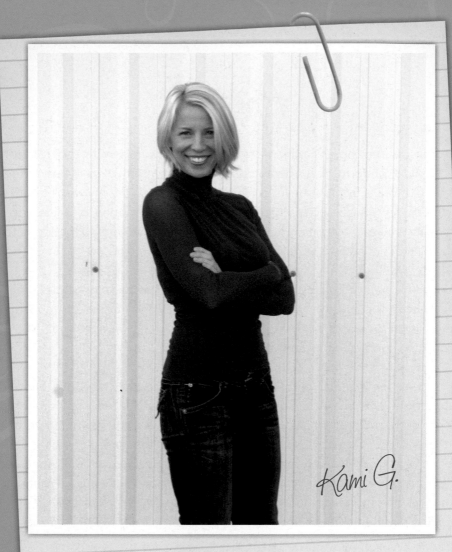

Kami G.

AGE:	43
HEIGHT:	5'6"
WEIGHT:	124 lbs
DRESS SIZE:	2/4
# OF CHILDREN:	2
PROFESSION:	TV wardrobe stylist, author, style and image consultant

Kami G.

My jeans used to be six sizes larger than they are today. Then I had an epiphany about how my weight was directly related to unwholesome eating habits (duh!), so I made an instantaneous and concerted effort to consume only real foods. Slowly and steadily, I dropped the excess weight and returned to the size I was in high school. I'm still that size 23 years later.

I'm a habit-centered girl. I eat three meals (one is very light) and two snacks a day. So exactly what do I eat? I eat real, whole foods such as unrefined whole grains, legumes, lentils, fruits, vegetables, low-fat dairy, eggs, lean meats or seafood, and good fats like olives, nuts, and seeds. For a snack I have string cheese, raw nuts, and fruit. There are many things that I don't eat such as refined and processed foods or anything containing additives such as fat-free, diet, or light-packaged items, anything containing high-fructose corn syrup, artificial sweeteners, and trans-fats. For the occasional sweetener, I go for unrefined, low-glycemic substitutes such as maple syrup, agave nectar, or brown rice syrup. Even on my birthday, I take a pass on cake! For dinner I stick to a deck-of-card-sized portions, make it my last meal of the day, and never have dessert. I supplement with fish oil to ensure I'm getting enough in the way of essential fatty acids.

For exercise, I walk everywhere and throw in the occasional Pilates class. And being a stylist means I'm a bag-schlepper, which has given me very strong biceps!

I never weigh myself, but when my jeans feel snug, I rein things in a bit, and return to my über-healthy eating habits!

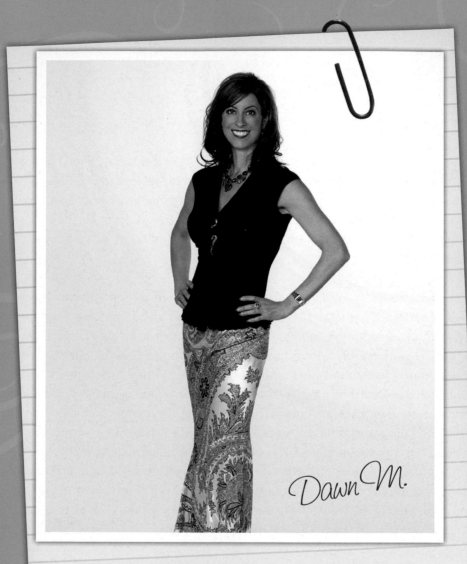

Dawn M.

AGE:	44
HEIGHT:	5'8"
WEIGHT:	I don't believe in scales
DRESS SIZE:	4
PROFESSION:	spiritual intuitive, expansion and beauty consciousness expert

Dawn M.

As a child, I was what one might describe as pleasantly plump. However, today I eat healthily, concentrating on getting enough protein in conjunction with limiting simple carbohydrates and fat intake. I allow myself one day each week to enjoy whatever I desire, and as a result, I don't feel deprived. I listen to my body by eating when it is hungry and stopping when full, and found I can easily maintain my weight this way.

I drink at least three glasses of water daily, I take a multivitamin, omega-3, calcium, vitamin D, a powder antioxidant blend, and a supplement by Greens for the abs.

I exercise at home five days per week, doing 30 minutes of aerobics combined with weight training. Beachbody's *ChaLEAN® Extreme* is my favorite program, as well as power yoga, which strengthens my core and keeps me flexible.

It is a challenge to stay fit, but one that I embrace due to my desire to feel healthy, vibrant, and strong. My daily routine also includes meditation, which contributes to my feeling balanced and calm. As within, so without!

"It is a challenge to stay fit, but one that I embrace."

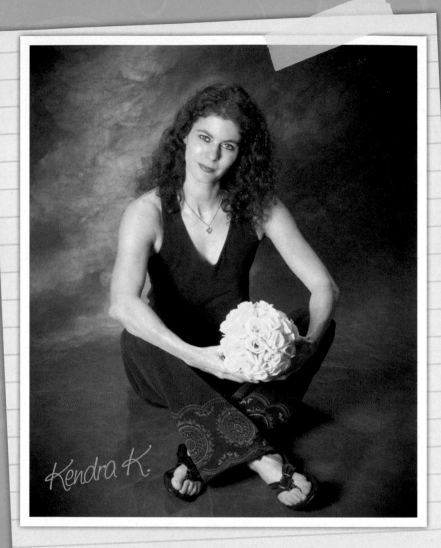

Kendra K.

AGE:	44
HEIGHT:	5'6"
WEIGHT:	112 lbs
DRESS SIZE:	4
# OF CHILDREN:	1
PROFESSION:	entrepreneur/product designer, mom, special events professional

Kendra K.

Growing up I avoided physical activity—I was your typical girly-girl! However, in college I took up weight training and running, and caught the fitness bug! It was only when I reached my 30's that I started thinking about exercise as a form of health insurance. Today I prefer less-impactful activities such as the elliptical machine, cross-trainer, and stationary bike.

Today I am conscious of maintaining a healthy diet. I eat three main meals a day, plus a couple of snacks. Breakfast is a bowl of whole-grain cereal with raisins and skim milk. Then I have fruit, cheese, or half a whole-wheat bagel as a mid-morning snack. Lunch is a lean protein on wheat bread, followed by a piece of fruit or the occasional juice. Dinner is grilled chicken, pasta, or brown rice and veggies. I avoid processed foods and supplement with a multivitamin, flax seed oil, and lutein for eye health.

I hit the gym four to five times a week for a minimum of 30 minutes of aerobics followed by a bit of weight training.

The above regimen of carefully chosen foods plus regular exercise helps me maintain a healthy body. And as a result, I hardly ever think about my weight, which is very liberating!

"I avoid processed foods."

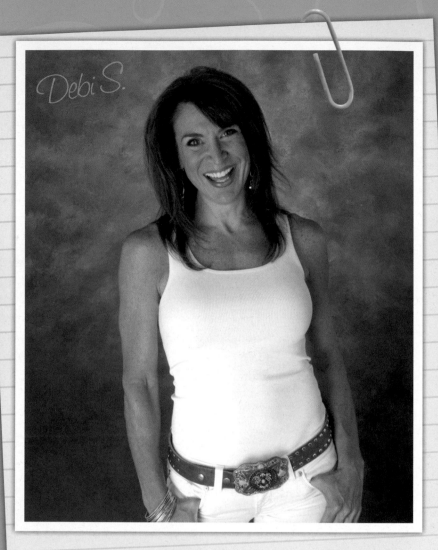

AGE: 44

HEIGHT: 5'5"

WEIGHT: 122 lbs

DRESS SIZE: 4

OF CHILDREN: 4

PROFESSION: dietitian, personal trainer,
health coach, author

Debi S.

What can I say? I love food! I have a healthy appetite and can gain weight easily. So when I'm fit, it's because I'm consciously working on my eating, exercise, and lifestyle habits. No mystery there!

I eat three meals and two snacks a day. Breakfast is a protein bar or a variety of healthy cereals mixed together, followed by yogurt as a mid-morning snack. Lunch is a large salad with fish, beans, nuts, eggs, seeds, and perhaps a bit of cheese. An afternoon snack is veggies with dip, fruit, nuts, whole-grain crackers, or cereal with soy milk. Simple carbs give me energy and sure taste good, but to my dismay, cause weight gain. Therefore, I pair them with a protein such as peanut butter, cottage cheese, or a handful of nuts, which provides me with a feeling of satisfaction. Dinner is a whole grain, veggies and beans, nuts, or seafood. I also drink water throughout the day, sometimes flavoring it with Crystal Light for added zing.

Exercise is my number-one stress reliever and keeps me fit and toned. I run or go to the gym to use the stair climber or elliptical machine. I also incorporate free weights, a universal machine, or resistance bands. Sometimes I just stay home and put on an exercise video. I step on the scale only occasionally, preferring to judge my weight simply by how my clothes fit.

For me, being in shape is like putting on a great pair of heels—it simply gives me that extra boost of mojo! I didn't say it was easy—far from it. But worth the effort? No doubt about it!

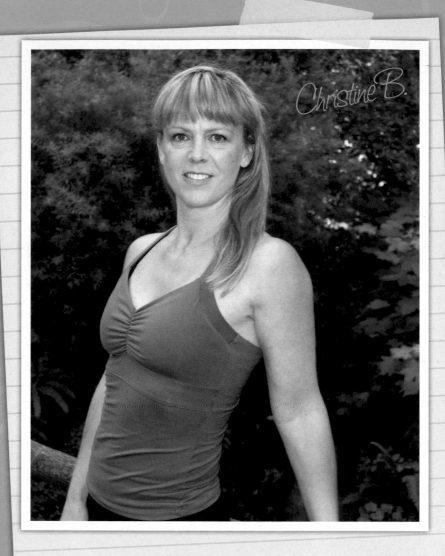

Christine B.

AGE: 44
HEIGHT: 5'8"
WEIGHT: 155 lbs
DRESS SIZE: 6
PROFESSION: author, Pilates professional

Christine B.

Staying active in ways that I enjoy is key to my health and fitness. For example, I live near a park with miles of walking, hiking, and running trails. I find that the amount of movement I do is more important than speed when it comes to energy and weight maintenance. Therefore, my aim is 10,000 steps per day, which can be either quick or leisurely.

Today I eat a small meal every three hours. My staples include vegetables, lean protein, and good fats such as non-fat Greek yogurt with fresh fruit and a sprinkle of nuts, an egg-white frittata with veggies, salad, beef with broccoli, and non-fat cottage cheese with fruit. I love teas of all kinds such as green, rooibos, and ginger, which packs an antioxidant punch that boosts the immune system. I stay away from sugars, preservatives, and chemicals. My secret weapons are supplements recommended by a naturopath: bio-identical hormones, maca root for energy, co-enzyme Q10, and vitamin D. These beauties have helped even out the hormonal roller coaster!

Pilates is a passion for me, an activity I truly enjoy! In addition, I include five hours of muscle building and flexibility training per week. I carry more muscle than your average gal, which keeps me slim and allows me to eat more.

Between maintaining a healthy diet and a regular exercise program, I feel well-balanced. I listen to my body, and it usually tells me what's best for it!

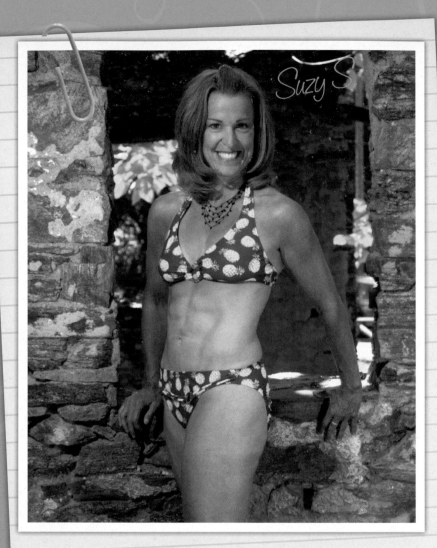

AGE:	45
HEIGHT:	5'6"
WEIGHT:	135 lbs
DRESS SIZE:	4/6
# OF CHILDREN:	3
PROFESSION:	mom, fitness coach, trainer

Suzy S.

I struggled with my weight for as long as I can remember. I went to the gym constantly, but never got the results I was looking for. Before finding an exercise program that worked for me, my state of mind was that of a frumpy middle-aged woman, yet I wanted to feel and look great for my age. One day I saw a P90X® infomercial. I was skeptical at first, but felt inspired enough to try something new. Every three months I took my picture and was shocked at the results. In 90 days I went down three sizes and entirely reshaped my body—it worked better than two decades of going to a gym!

I also made healthy dietary choices and continue to do so. For example, I eat five to six small meals throughout the day, and use a meal-replacement shake (Beachbody's Shakeology®) to manage my weight. I drink six to eight glasses of water a day and supplement with the basics such as omega-3, calcium, and a high-quality multivitamin.

I work out an hour a day to maintain my fitness, constantly changing up my routines to keep my body guessing and avoid hitting a plateau. I now have great abs and best of all, I can walk on the beach in a bikini!

I was not truly comfortable in my own skin until P90X transformed my body, and ultimately, my life. The feelings of well-being I receive from my daily commitment to exercise have spilled over into other aspects of my life as well. For example, I no longer think about food or my weight, and as a result, I feel younger and better than ever before. I have achieved total body confidence and it feels fabulous!

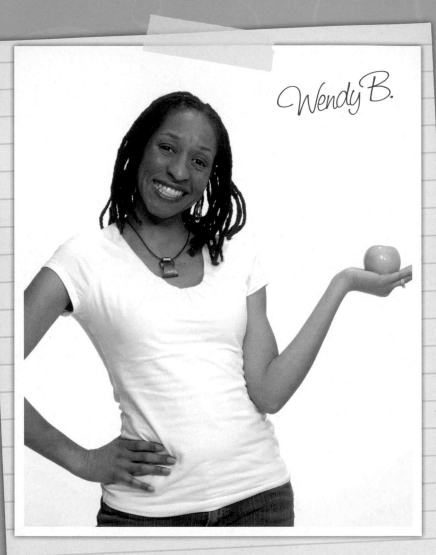

Wendy B.

AGE: 45

HEIGHT: 5'3"

WEIGHT: 120 lbs

DRESS SIZE: 4

PROFESSION: nutritionist, health coach

Wendy B.

Growing up, I wasn't so good at most things athletic. I felt redeemed when Jane Fonda came along with her workout videos—finally something that didn't involve a team or interacting with a ball! But when I went to college, it didn't take long to outgrow my clothes thanks to late night snacking and woefully small amounts of exercise.

Today I eat very moderately and pay attention to tasting and enjoying my meals. I subscribe to the clean eating lifestyle, emphasizing whole foods like fruits, veggies, and whole grains, and I steer clear of processed foods. I use fresh herbs, a variety of spices, natural sweeteners, and minimal amounts of salt. I drink eight glasses of water a day as well. This gives me a good indication of when I'm full, helps avoid overeating, and minimizes sugar cravings.

When it comes to exercise, I walk during the nice weather, and belong to a gym during cooler months. I do cardio a couple times a week as well as weight lifting. It's a fantastic means to ignite fat burning, and keeps my bones strong to boot.

I'm not a calorie counter but I do weigh the ramifications before choosing certain foods. For me, self-awareness is key to a positive outlook on life, maintaining a healthy weight, and feeling good in my body!

"I use fresh herbs, a variety of spices, natural sweeteners."

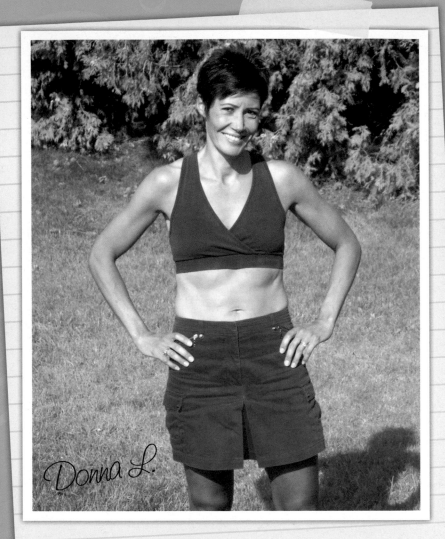

Donna L.

AGE: 45
HEIGHT: 5'8"
WEIGHT: 125 lbs
DRESS SIZE: 6
OF CHILDREN: 3
PROFESSION: mortgage broker

Donna L.

I was always a skinny kid, until one day Aunt Bea came to visit and brought chocolate, which I started eating for breakfast! This habit caused me to gain unsightly fat during high school. I tried dieting, but it was always accompanied by frustrating amounts of deprivation. But what finally turned me around was education. I learned that eating five small meals a day was instrumental in weight loss. The best part about this approach was that as soon as I started feeling hungry, I knew I'd soon be eating again—no starving allowed!

Today I stick to healthy snacks such as fruit and nuts between meals, and I stay away from unnecessary simple carbs. My home is full of nature-created items such as butter, milk, coconut oil, eggs, and meat as opposed to genetically-altered substances such as margarine, liquid eggs, and fat-free milk. I also stay away from soda and processed foods. I learned that healthy fats (such as coconut oil) are very good for the body and have been shown to aid in weight loss. I supplement with calcium, vitamin C, omega-3, and a good probiotic.

My exercise program consists of weight training twice a week and cardiovascular interval training two to three times per week. I've learned that for fat loss (which is more readily gained as life goes on), weight training is really important as cardio alone seldom does the trick. I always drink plenty of water while working out.

I notice that when I'm eating properly (i.e., limiting sugar and white-flour products), my clothes continue to fit just fine. It's only when I've consumed too many simple carbs that I observe changes in my body. Therefore, I make a lifestyle choice to watch what I eat and pay attention to how much activity I can fit in. As a result, I look forward to good health as I approach the half-century mark, and am proud of the body that I have!

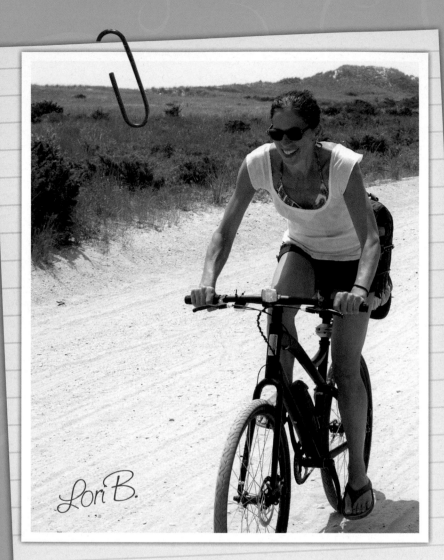

Lori B.

AGE:	46
HEIGHT:	5'6"
WEIGHT:	124 lbs
DRESS SIZE:	4
PROFESSION:	actor, writer, musician

Lori B.

As a child I was encouraged to be active, and grew up with good eating habits. My parents kept a watchful eye on sugar consumption, and my great-grandfather from Italy instilled the philosophy that moderation was the key to life.

Today I eat local, organic food. I also incorporate many things into my lifestyle that I learned from Deepak Chopra's book *Perfect Health,* which focuses on the ancient Ayurvedic system to achieve optimum body and mind, based on prevention and a person's individual constitution. Technically a pescetarian, I eat three meals a day and in between I have little snacks to keep my energy up. I enjoy many kinds of greens and vegetables, beans, tofu, whole fruits, and nuts, and occasionally fish. I stay away from anything with white sugar, and rarely have soda, but do enjoy the occasional alcoholic beverage. If I eat bread it will be of the multi-grain or whole-wheat variety. I drink five to six glasses of water per day and enjoy green tea in the afternoon. I supplement with a multivitamin, a B-complex, vitamin D, and vitamin C.

I start every day with stretching or yoga, followed by a three-to-four mile run twice a week. When the weather is warmer, I bike, rollerblade, and swim.

I believe that moderation, as well as taking care of my body by eating well and exercising, are the keys to keeping me healthy and toned in both body and mind.

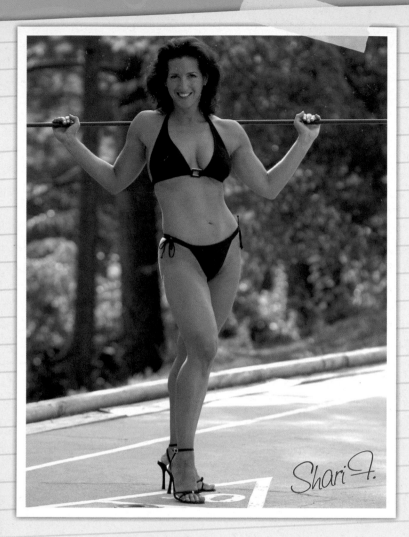

Shari F.

AGE: 46

HEIGHT: 5'2"

WEIGHT: 115 lbs

DRESS SIZE: 2

PROFESSION: certified fitness professional, certified specialist in fitness nutrition, natural health advocate

Shari F.

I used to ogle "before" and "after" transformation pictures in fitness magazines. Personally, I was frustrated, frumpy, and a perpetual "before" picture. It wasn't as if I wasn't trying—heck, I practically lived at the gym! And I thought I was eating healthy, so for the life of me, I couldn't figure out what I was doing wrong! Discontent finally led me to investigate what some of the top experts in the fitness industry had to say. I started keeping a journal of my diet and workouts, and it wasn't long before I was able to see the mistakes I was making.

My biggest error was that I was eating too many of the wrong carbohydrates and not enough lean protein or the right fats. Another mistake was that I was doing too much cardio and not enough strength training. My body had become a fat-*storing* instead of a fat-*burning* machine! I applied the information I was learning, and from making a few simple changes, my body began transforming. I never dreamed that I would achieve such dramatic results!

Making over my body from fat and flabby to fit, healthy, and toned took commitment and didn't happen overnight. However, overall it was by far an easy process, and one that anyone can achieve with the right tools. Today I have a high lean-muscle to body-fat ratio and I'm healthier than ever before. Never in my wildest dreams did I ever think I would be a real-life success story! I am a living example that healthy eating habits and consistent strength training can truly lead to the fountain of youth!

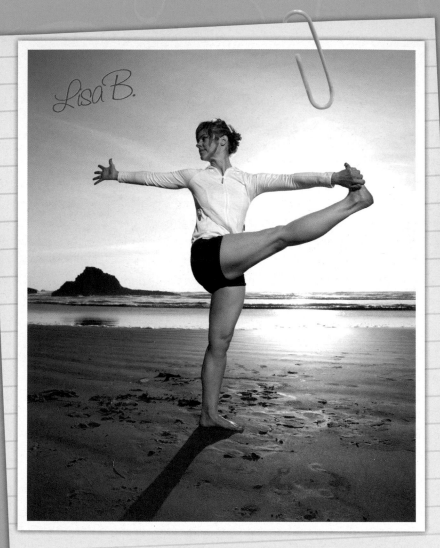

Lisa B.

AGE:	46
HEIGHT:	5'7"
WEIGHT:	128 lbs
DRESS SIZE:	6
PROFESSION:	yoga teacher

Lisa B.

Growing up, I loved playing outdoors. Then in high school, I became somewhat of a vegetarian, and learned the importance of vitamin supplementation. After graduation, I unexpectedly put on a few pounds, so I started running in an attempt to take off the weight. It worked wonders, so I kept it up.

Today there are a couple of things I don't eat: wheat and processed sugar. I totally avoid fast food or anything packaged, processed, or frozen. I keep my weight stable by staying aware of when I feel full, so as to not overeat. I also drink plenty of water.

I practice yoga four to five times a week and walk instead of drive when distance permits.

On the whole, I pay more attention to how I feel than the way I look. And for this, I would have to credit my yoga practice for being instrumental in helping me see my life in a more complete and healthier light!

"I keep my weight stable by staying aware of when I feel full, so as to not overeat."

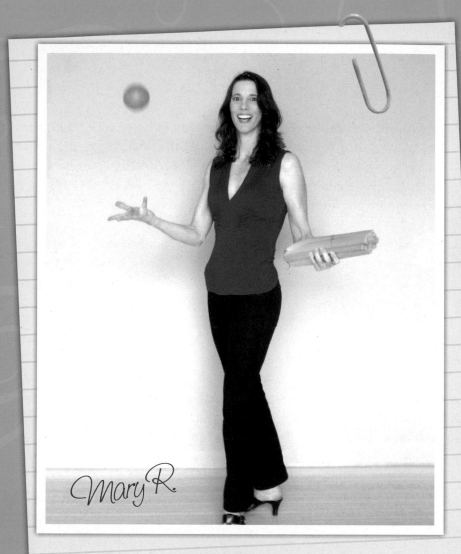

Mary R.

AGE:	47
HEIGHT:	5'10"
WEIGHT:	130 lbs
DRESS SIZE:	4
# OF CHILDREN:	3
PROFESSION:	healthy-eating expert

Mary R.

During my college years, if I did a good job studying (or even a bad job) of studying, I would reward myself with my favorite sweet treat. The result? I gained weight—and a lot of it! I knew I needed a healthier diet, but it wasn't until I had children that I realized devouring pie à la mode did not make me feel more successful, beautiful, or more satisfied. I just felt stuffed full of pie!

Today I use non-food rewards for a job well done, such as a fun crossword puzzle or a book. I focus on eating colorful, fresh foods, making sure to eat every three hours, or five times a day with a little protein at each meal, controlling my portion sizes by eating on small plates. I also follow three simple rules:

1. Eat breakfast every day.
2. Run away from partially-hydrogenated vegetable oil (trans-fats).
3. Avoid high-fructose corn syrup (corn sugar) like the plague.

To keep active, I swim three days a week, and I am delighted that I can now put on a bikini instead of my usual one-piece!

For me, looking good is about creating a healthy relationship with food. I make healthy choices every day, because as I finally learned, I am worth it.

"I focus on eating colorful, fresh foods."

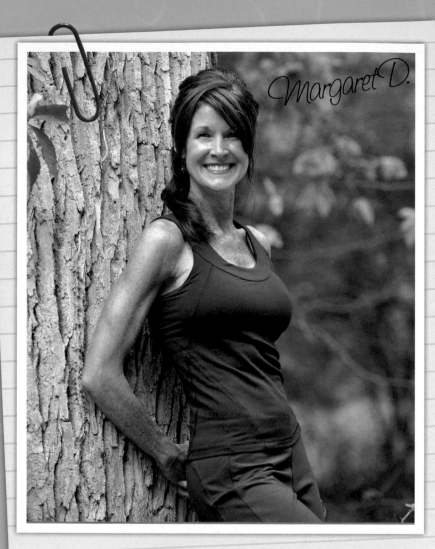

Margaret D.

AGE:	47
HEIGHT:	5'8"
WEIGHT:	122 lbs
DRESS SIZE:	0/2
# OF CHILDREN:	2
PROFESSION:	healthcare marketing and sales professional

Margaret D.

I have been thin most of my life, but not always fit. So after having children, I decided to get into shape and include weight training (which was the turning point in getting me really fit). I learned effective and efficient exercise habits, as well as the value of proper nutrition and the role it plays in maintaining a healthy weight.

Ideally, I eat a protein and healthy carb every few hours. I start the morning with a cup of tea with honey or agave to sweeten, followed by egg whites and fibrous foods such as oatmeal and cereal, to which I add a scoop of protein powder. I enjoy Mediterranean foods such as grape leaves, tabouli, hummus, and fava bean salad, and I eat a lot of avocados, raw nuts, and fruits and veggies such as spinach, peppers, tomatoes, apples, oranges, and berries. I also include dairy such as eggs, organic skim milk, and yogurt, as well as a variety of lean meats. I enjoy high-fiber pasta and bread in moderation, such as pizza on a whole-wheat crust maybe once or twice per month. I do not eat fast or fried foods, chips, doughnuts, or pastries, or drink soda, sports drinks, fruit juice, or coffee, and make a point of wrapping up my eating by 7 p.m. I drink five to six glasses of water a day as well.

I exercise for 45 to 50 minutes every morning before I eat, beginning with a 20-minute cardio interval workout. Mixing it up is key, so I alternate between the treadmill, stationary bike, elliptical machine, and Stairmaster. I train with weights and do abdominal crunches using a ball, machine, or a combination of the two. I end the day with a 20-minute walk, rain or shine.

I like the way my clothes fit, so if I feel my jeans getting snug, I simply work out harder or walk a little extra until everything feels comfortable again, and I'm back to feeling my best!

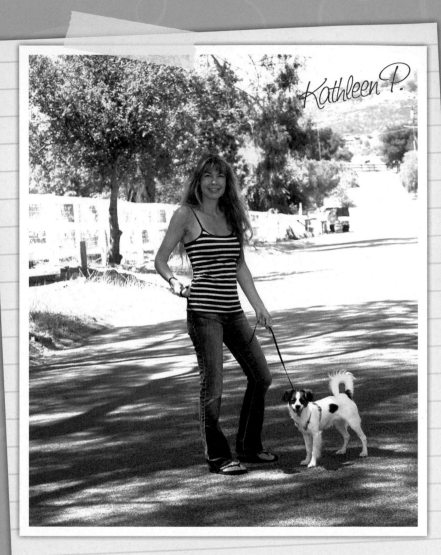

Kathleen P.

AGE:	47
HEIGHT:	5'5"
WEIGHT:	112 lbs
DRESS SIZE:	2/4
# OF CHILDREN:	3
PROFESSION:	holistic health practitioner

Kathleen P.

Although I have always been slender, I thoroughly enjoy food! However, I pay attention to being present with my meals by eating without distractions. I chew my food well, consume balanced snacks, stop eating when I'm full, and make sure to have something small as soon as I feel hungry. In this way, I feel satisfied.

I eat three times a day, concentrating on organic and seasonal foods that grow in my area. I am careful not to skip a meal, and when I snack, I have protein, a healthy carb, and some fat to balance digestion and to keep my energy levels even. I never eat carbohydrates alone. And when I feel hungry I may drink some water and wait a couple of minutes. If I'm still hungry, I know it is time to eat. (Sometimes, you're just thirsty.) I like a flat stomach, so I avoid wheat. I don't drink soda as this can also contribute to a bloated stomach. I don't drink juice without fiber because my body starts to look for it by sending hunger signals. I also avoid alcohol and coffee, preferring to sip water throughout the day.

I enjoy outdoor exercise such as walking and hiking. I also stretch and practice yoga, and love to dance.

I believe I stay slim because of healthy fats, such as butter and coconut oil, which seems a bit contradictory, but they actually help to burn fat. It's the simple carbs that contribute to a buildup of fat in the system and throughout the body. So I simply avoid those foods and go on my merry way. Because of these principles I am usually taken for much younger than I actually am and I feel great. How cool is that?

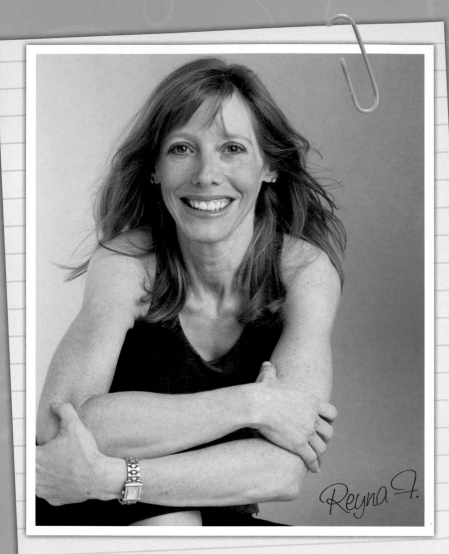

Reyna F.

AGE: 47

HEIGHT: 5'1"

WEIGHT: 99 lbs

DRESS SIZE: 0

OF CHILDREN: 1

PROFESSION: registered dietitian,
certified personal trainer

Reyna T.

My weight has remained fairly stable throughout my life. This is probably due to the fact that I eat healthfully, enjoy going to the gym, and love outdoor sports and activities.

I eat every three to four hours to fuel my body and mind. For breakfast, I have whole-grain cereal, nonfat milk, and a piece of fruit followed by a mid-morning snack that combines protein and carbs. Lunch may be a veggie burger with lettuce, tomato, and whole-wheat bread. Then I have a midday snack of string cheese, nuts, fruit, or yogurt. Dinner is fish, tofu, or beans with a whole grain and vegetables. I use a small plate to control my portions, and pay attention to when I'm full—and then stop eating. I drink water throughout the day, and if I get hungry at night, I have a protein shake. I also take vitamin D and a fish-oil supplement.

During the warmer months, I run, bike, ski, hike, and rock climb. During winter months I ski, run, or go to the gym for cardio and/or strength training. I drink water when exercising, adding in a bit of carbohydrate/electrolyte replacement for stamina if my exercise is longer than 90 minutes.

I enjoy a healthy lifestyle. I like the way exercising makes me look and feel, so I don't consider it a chore. Exercise energizes me, which I believe is an essential key to life, along with whole foods, friends, family, and the outdoors.

"I eat every three to four hours to fuel my body and mind."

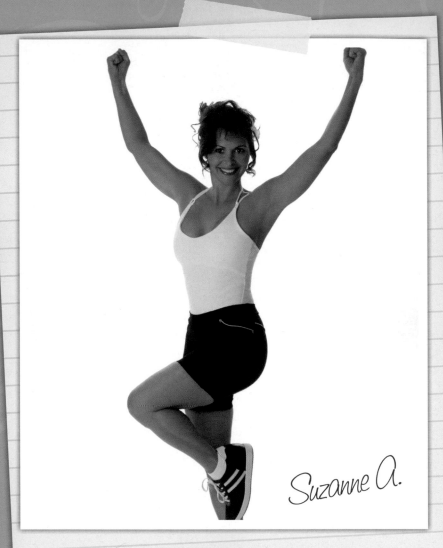

Suzanne A.

AGE:	47
HEIGHT:	5'2"
WEIGHT:	115 lbs
DRESS SIZE:	4/6
# OF CHILDREN:	1
PROFESSION:	TV fitness host

Suzanne A.

After I gave birth, I couldn't see my toes. The simple act of walking was an arduous task and every step was excruciating. A friend told me about how meditation could benefit me. I was skeptical, since at first I didn't understand how a sedentary activity could help me lose weight. However, I was open to learning, and it was not long before I discovered the secret—that during meditation, my mind is the boss and my body is the dutiful employee. I tell my body what it needs to do and it follows suit! And the same, breathing techniques I used to control my appetite and regulate stress also helped me develop my lungs. Today I feel energized to exercise, make healthy dietary choices, and control my portion sizes.

I practice gentle yoga combined with low-impact exercises. This not only helps keep the pounds off, but also makes day-to-day tasks more manageable. I also combine low-impact techniques with high-intensity workouts, and in this way, have successfully turned my body from a fat-storing machine into an automated fat-burning one!

Meditation motivates me to lose the excuses so that I stay on track. I credit my weight-loss accomplishment to the reflection of mind, body, and spirit. I participate actively in my healthcare plan by using preventative, cost-effective approaches to managing my overall wellness: a good, healthy diet and a solid, consistent commitment to exercise. I am the CEO of my health and I have never felt better!

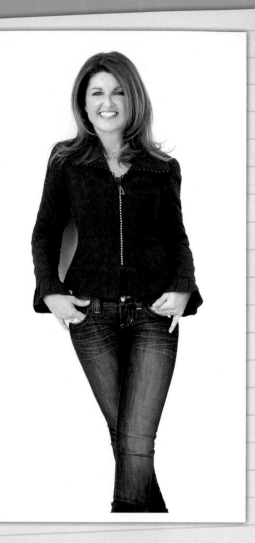

Kelly B.

AGE:	47
HEIGHT:	5'1"
WEIGHT:	I would rather give you my PIN
DRESS SIZE:	2
# OF CHILDREN:	3
PROFESSION:	success coach and trainer, motivational speaker

Kelly B.

I never had a weight problem, so calorie count and nutrition weren't even a thought—that is, until after my first pregnancy when I gained four sizes! Out of sheer anxiety, I started paying close attention to nutrition and exercise, reading everything I possibly could on the subject. After I had my son, I had to get to work real fast on losing the remaining 30 pounds! I had a six-week follow-up with my doctor and I wanted to make sure I fit into my pre-pregnancy jeans. Jane Fonda was the craze at that time and that's all I did. I counted calories and worked out with Jane every day! I fit back into those jeans and have kept the fit lifestyle ever since.

Today I enjoy a vegetarian diet and eat only when I'm hungry. For breakfast I have an egg-white omelet with peppers or whole-wheat toast and peanut butter. Mid-morning I have a fruit smoothie with Vega Blend, a plant-based protein formula for energy. Lunch is a vegetarian sandwich, green tea, and the occasional organic ginger snap as a treat. I love, love, love Thai food, so that is usually dinner: rice or pad Thai pasta with vegetables and tofu. I also drink plenty of water and love my tea!

Today I work out like crazy! It is my favorite thing to do. I get up at six and get on the Stairmaster for an hour doing 10.76 miles. I need this for energy. If I don't work out, I feel tired and crabby. I mix in FIRM workouts and Cathe Friedrich a few times a week. Weather permitting, I trade the Stairmaster workout for running. One thing that I won't do is step onto a scale; I just make sure that my clothes fit properly.

When I have a healthy lifestyle, it spills into other areas of my life. I'm glad to stay fit because last year I ran my first full marathon and absolutely loved it!

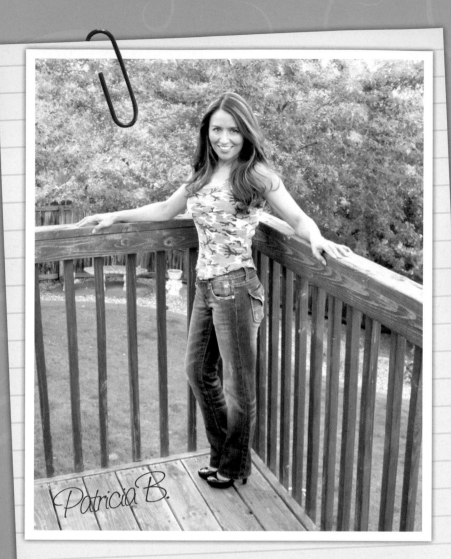

Patricia B.

AGE:	48
HEIGHT:	4'11"
WEIGHT:	98 lbs
DRESS SIZE:	1
# OF CHILDREN	2
PROFESSION:	realtor

Patricia B.

When I was younger it was easy to control my weight; if I put on a couple of pounds I'd fast for a day and be right back where I was. But today, I really have to work at it by watching everything I eat. And because it is important for me to stay slim, everything I do revolves around how not to gain weight. I stick to eating right, exercising, and striving to have a good attitude at all times.

Today I adhere to the following philosophy: eat breakfast like a king, lunch like a prince, and dinner like a pauper. I keep my metabolism high by eating small things all day like celery sticks with cheese, nuts, fruits, and all kinds of salads with anything that is in season. If ice cream, cookies, and chocolate are in the house, chances are I am going to indulge, so I don't buy them. Pizza is my weakness, so after the occasional slice I balance it by running an extra mile or two the next day. I avoid white bread, potatoes, and rice, and never eat past 7 p.m. I supplement with calcium.

For exercise, I have a gym membership and a treadmill, and do at least three miles of walking or running a day. Also, I enjoy turning daily things into exercise such as walking the dog, raking the leaves, and shoveling the snow. Or I park away from my destination a bit so I have longer to walk.

I think about my weight all the time as for me, being thin is a constant day-by-day battle. My motto: *If I don't look good, I don't feel good*. Although staying in shape is a lot of work, it's worth it!

"Fitness—if it came in a bottle, everybody would have a great body!"

~Cher

The 50's

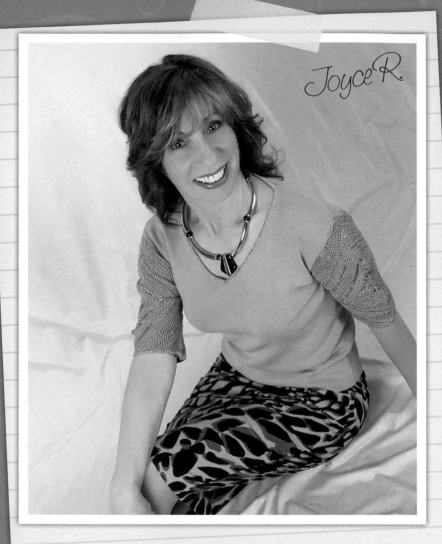

Joyce R.

AGE: 50+

HEIGHT: 5'2"

WEIGHT: 119 lbs

DRESS SIZE: 4

OF CHILDREN: 2

PROFESSION: writing consultant

Joyce R.

I was never overweight until I worked at a desk all day. Kind friends attributed it to middle age spread—something I should accept because "that's what happens when you get older." At first, I bought into it. After all, my mother was obese; therefore, I was doomed! Fat was in my DNA; I might as well accept it and move on, right? But something deep inside me refused to believe this. Determined to defy conventional wisdom, I joined Weight Watchers, and over time, conventional wisdom was indeed defied! To this day, I still practice what I learned. Food choices and portion control are only half of my four-pronged approach. The other two are exercise and awareness.

Today, I eat three meals and two snacks a day. I include protein in each meal—including breakfast—and peanuts, pistachios, or hummus with fresh vegetables are my munchies of choice. Before Weight Watchers, prepared and processed foods were part of the menu. Today, dinners consist of lean protein such as chicken breast, top round, or pork tenderloin; salads are dark, leafy greens and tomatoes, and instead of bottled dressing, olive oil and balsamic vinegar. I cut back on starchy potatoes, white rice, and pasta. If I do have pasta, it's whole wheat only. Portion control also plays a big part in my dietary approach: I know how much food is in a serving, and I rarely go for a seconds. And for dessert? It's fresh fruit when it's in season. Sweet treats like cake, cookies, and ice cream are no longer in the house. And I take fish oil and a multivitamin to supplement my diet.

I run four to six miles, three times a week, and lift weights once or twice a week. And to stay on track, I weigh myself every couple of days.

The bottom line is that I believe in choices. Although it takes awareness and hard work, I choose with purpose because of the overall sense of well-being it brings me. As a result, I'm a smaller, happier, and more energetic person!

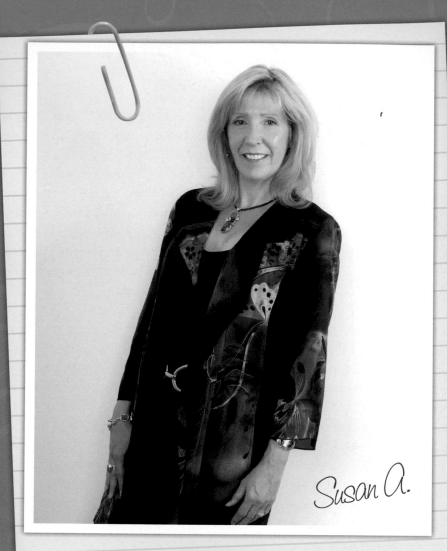

Susan A.

AGE:	50
HEIGHT:	5'3"
WEIGHT:	115 lbs
DRESS SIZE:	2
# OF CHILDREN:	2 stepsons
PROFESSION:	speaker, trainer, personal development expert

Susan A.

As a teen I rocked a boyish figure. My mother used to say I'd be glad later in life to be able to eat anything and never gain weight. That proved to be the case, that is, until I turned forty, when I could no longer indulge without consequences! Not knowing too much about nutrition, diets, or exercise, I started to ask questions. A colleague told me if I drank a lot of water, I would flush fat-storing toxins, so I started drinking six to eight glasses a day. I also started lifting weights a bit. In an effort to avoid sabotaging my hard work, I cut out simple sugars—at least the kind found in junk food. Within a few months I had lost all of the excess weight—hooray!

Today I eat three meals a day. Breakfast is yogurt and fruit or toast, lunch is soup or a healthy sandwich, and dinner consists of fish or chicken with salad or brown rice. When I'm traveling it's a whole different story, and there are dietary challenges that make vitamins quite important! I take a multivitamin to help balance hormones, as well as a B-complex and magnesium.

I exercise along with Pilates, yoga, weight training, and aerobic DVDs for 20–30 minutes, four days a week. When I travel I rely on walking, putting aside at least an hour a day.

I do not step on a scale that often, but I don't feel comfortable when my weight gets past a certain point so I'm careful about what I consume. If I crave something other than healthy things, I partake, but in moderation. Yes, the balance of diet and exercise sounds so cliché, but it works for me and I'm not about to reinvent the wheel!

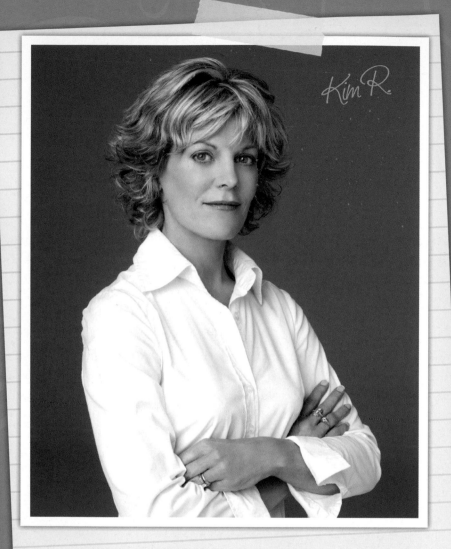

Kim R.

AGE: 51

HEIGHT: 5'6"

WEIGHT: 110 lbs

DRESS SIZE: 4

OF CHILDREN: 2

PROFESSION: writer, wife, mother, animal wrangler

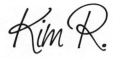

Kim R.

I've always been thin. However, I concentrate on healthy meals and limit fatty foods when cooking.

I've been a longtime connoisseur of peanut butter. Many years ago I came across a study that praised its health benefits, stating that it lowered bad and raised good cholesterol. As well as having great antioxidant content, peanut butter includes vitamin E, folic acid, and fiber, which are known to provide heart-disease protection. As an added benefit, I find it keeps my hunger at bay longer than some other low-fat, high-carbohydrate foods.

In terms of exercise, years ago, my husband gave me the gift of a few sessions with a personal trainer. It surpassed diamonds, chocolate, and flowers. It was just like the Visa commercial—priceless! My personal trainer showed me invaluable breathing techniques as well as how to do cardio and properly exercise with weights. He also taught me to incorporate stairs and chairs—things I already had in my home so I didn't need to buy expensive machines. My only investment was a cheap set of dumbbells purchased at my local discount store—a great deal for the thrifty mom!

My weight rarely fluctuates, and I believe it is the result of consistent workouts, along with a sensible and nutritious diet. In this way I am able to maintain my small frame, and feel energetic and healthy overall.

"I concentrate on healthy meals and limit fatty foods when cooking."

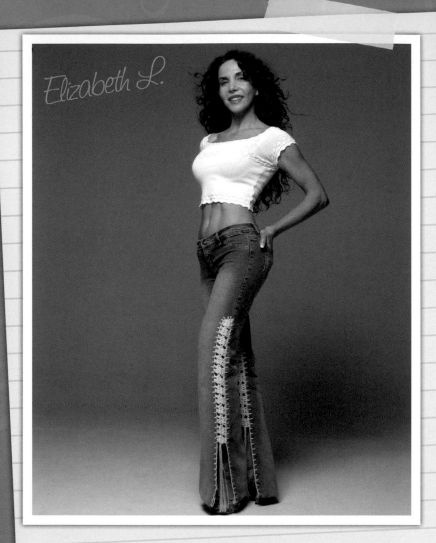

Elizabeth L.

AGE: 51

HEIGHT: 5'4"

WEIGHT: 105 lbs

DRESS SIZE: 2

PROFESSION: inspirational speaker, talk show host; vitality, vibrancy, and youthfulness expert

Elizabeth L.

People might say that I was just naturally thin growing up, but that is not necessarily true. I have been disciplined about eating and exercising since adolescence and I have always been interested in health, fitness, and nutrition. By the time I was in high school, I began treating my body like an experimental lab in an effort to discover which foods yielded me the most strength and energy.

My philosophy today is to put living foods into my body. I have eliminated all processed foods—I eat predominantly raw—and as a result, I experience a tremendous life force, light, and vitality.

I am passionate about fitness, and enjoy discovering new and exciting ways to stay active. For example, I love everything from roller-skating to bungee jumping and tightrope walking! Dancing also gives me great joy and helps me maintain a youthful body, mind, and spirit.

For me, keeping fit is about adopting a lifestyle consciousness. What I eat, as well as how I move and think, are directly connected to my vibrancy and youthfulness, and allow me to experience overall health and well-being. As a result, I have become ageless, timeless, and limitless!

"Keeping fit is about adopting a lifestyle consciousness."

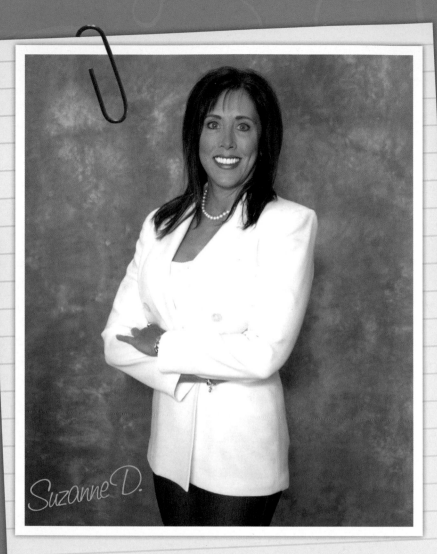

Suzanne D.

AGE:	52
HEIGHT:	5'5"
WEIGHT:	128 lbs
DRESS SIZE:	4
PROFESSION:	entrepreneur

Suzanne D.

Growing up, I was very thin, so I was able to eat whatever and whenever I wanted. I was also pretty active in gymnastics and softball throughout high school. Later on, when I started working full-time, I became involved with weightlifting and jogging, and as a result, I started to develop some shape—cool! I was firm, healthy, and clear-headed. In my mid-40's I started gaining weight! I soon found that paying attention to my eating habits and making time for exercise was crucial if I wanted to maintain the slim, sexy body I had become accustomed to!

Today, I pay attention to all of my meals. For example, I may have egg whites with cheese for breakfast, a big salad for lunch, and a piece of fish with steamed veggies for dinner. An evening snack is a handful of nuts or sugar-free ice cream.

I work out four to six times a week, changing it up to keep my muscles guessing. For example, on any given week, I may alternate between going to the gym and doing the elliptical machine, doing lunges and arm curls with lightweights while on a phone conference, or simply taking a jog around the block. This way I never get bored and look forward to keeping active!

"I soon found that paying attention to my eating habits and making time for exercise was crucial."

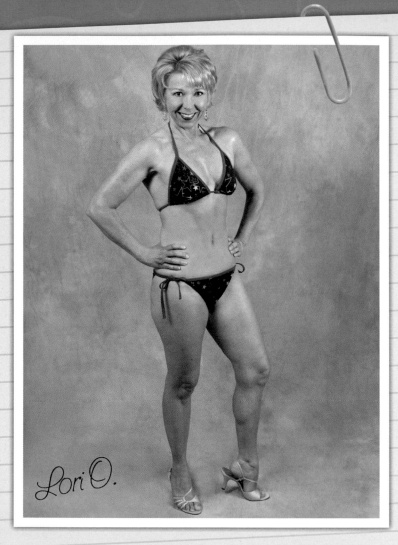

Lori O.

AGE:	51
HEIGHT:	5'2"
WEIGHT:	112 lbs
DRESS SIZE:	4
# OF CHILDREN:	2
PROFESSION:	CEO of an entertainment corporation, vocalist

Lori O.

I was about to hit mid-century and my weight was ballooning. Going through menopause didn't help matters, but I refused to use it as an excuse, so I decided to make some changes. My goal was to get my picture taken in a bikini for my 50th birthday! I got my blood work done, and on the advice of a doctor, got back in balance with bio-identical hormones: DHEA, Stress B Plus, Pregnenolone, Vitamin D, and Omega-3. In addition, I used Isagenix meal-replacement shakes and bars. Yet after losing an initial few pounds, I hit a plateau, and I soon learned that weight is hard to get and keep off without consistent exercise! So I joined a gym, but the real results came when I hired a personal trainer. My body made a dramatic transformation, something I had not been able to accomplish on my own.

Today I eat five to six small, 200-calorie meals a day, every two and a half hours. For breakfast, I have a vanilla-flavored whey protein shake with half a banana or Special K with skim milk, and blueberries for a snack. For lunch, I have two pieces of turkey breast with a slice of provolone, and an apple in the mid-afternoon. For dinner, I have chicken, rice, and vegetables, and frozen grapes for a nighttime snack. I also drink a lot Fuze Slenderize or water, often adding protein powder for flavor. I don't drink alcohol, coffee, fruit juice, or soda.

For exercise, I work out at home with P90X® at 7 a.m. every morning. It's intense, but I love it.

As a result of my efforts, my body is solid—the belly is gone and I'm in better shape than ever before!

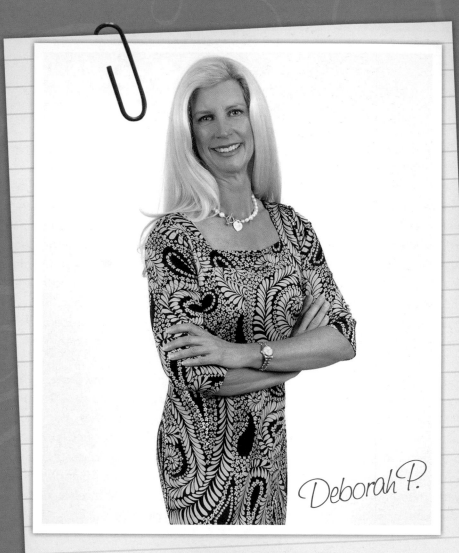

Deborah P.

AGE:	52
HEIGHT:	5'9"
WEIGHT:	128 lbs
DRESS SIZE:	4
# OF CHILDREN:	3
PROFESSION:	jewelry designer

Deborah P.

I spent most of my life overweight—from shopping at the chubby store as a kid to weighing over 200 pounds after having children. It was not long before I began to see the effects of my southern cooking on my little ones as well. So I started including salads at dinner and limiting the mashed potatoes, fried food, and biscuits. Gradually, as I substituted healthier foods in place of macaroni and cheese, hamburger helper, and meatloaf, I realized I had the power to change my own body as well!

Today I eat mostly organic. I gave up soda and fast food, not only because they are not good for my waistline, but also simply because they don't make me feel good. I drink up to eight glasses of water a day, and supplement with a multivitamin/mineral blend. On occasion I add an antioxidant mixture for skin health.

Every day, I run, do yoga, lift weights, or play golf. To avoid experiencing a plateau, I change things up a bit as soon as something feels easy.

One of my best motivational secrets is the technique of visualization. I cut out pictures of how I want to look, put them on a vision board, and compare myself to the photos. If I want to improve a certain body part, I concentrate on that area until I'm happy with the results. Today, I am proud to be maintaining these lifestyle changes long-term!

"Today I eat mostly organic."

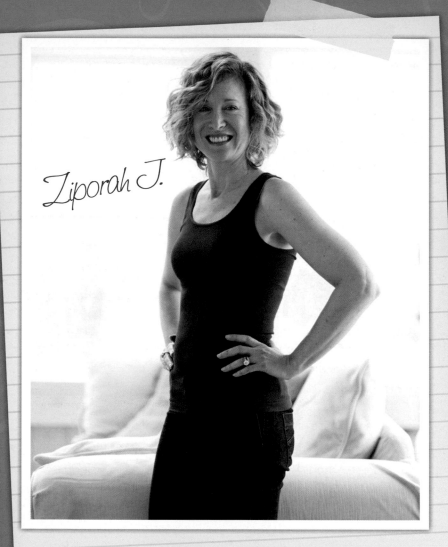

Ziporah J.

AGE: 52

HEIGHT: 5'4"

WEIGHT: 118 lbs

DRESS SIZE: 4

PROFESSION: lifestyle resort director

Ziporah J.

Growing up, I was a finicky eater, and therefore quite thin. In high school I kept active as a dancer, but after graduation gained some weight. It was then that I realized I couldn't eat whatever I wanted anymore without consequences. In order to maintain my figure, I set out to learn as much as I could about nutrition.

Today, I eat three meals a day and two snacks. I keep processed food out of the house, favoring grilled chicken, whole grains, and fresh fruit. I'm careful about portions: as long as I don't skip a meal and get too hungry, it's easy to keep portions reasonable. My formula is to eat protein, a bit of a healthy fat, and a good carb every three to four hours. I take a few supplements: calcium, vitamin D, folic acid, magnesium, and a multivitamin.

Other than walking my dog, I exercise a few times a week, such as taking a run, Pilates, yoga, or an aerobics class. And a few years back, a friend gave me a few sessions with a personal trainer. I loved it, so I continued on. That one hour a week has changed my physique, creating a well-toned look while strengthening my shoulders and abs. As another side benefit, my commitment to exercise has ultimately helped to successfully end a lifelong back strain.

The combination of exercising and eating a healthy diet truly does lead to the fountain of youth! No, staying active is not always easy, but I'd rather not experience the alternative. So I just do it, and joyfully!

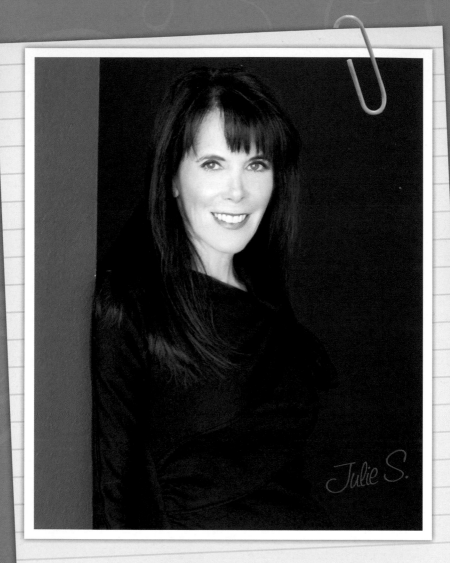

Julie S.

AGE:	52
HEIGHT:	5'3"
WEIGHT	104 lbs
DRESS SIZE:	2
PROFESSION:	author, dating coach, social media marketing executive

Julie S.

As a child I was very slight. My grandmother would bribe me with a dollar for every pound I gained while at summer camp. Entrepreneur that I was, I ate triple portions and made ten bucks every summer! Once back home, however, the weight would drop off again.

When I got to college, I ate fast food out of convenience. I was shocked to find myself four sizes larger at the end of my senior year! I tried every fad diet, but to no avail. Finally, I went with common sense. I eliminated sugar, bread, salt, and alcohol. I stopped eating after 7 p.m. I cut portions in half, eating the remainder at the next sitting. The result? In a few short months I had lost the weight.

Today, my exercise routine consists of Pilates twice a week and walking two to five miles on the weekends. When I notice the numbers on the scale tipping in the wrong direction, I go back to smaller portions, completely avoid sugar and carbs, and finish all eating by 7 p.m.

I weigh myself daily to keep things in check. I enjoy a bit of sugar and bread now and then, but do it in moderation. Portion control has been key for me in my efforts to stay slim.

"I enjoy a bit of sugar and bread now and then, but do it in moderation."

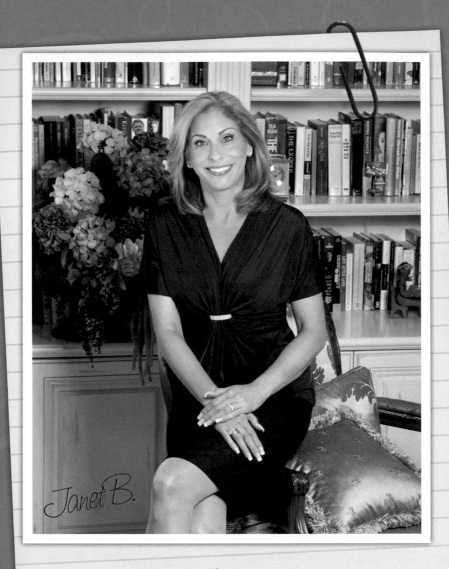

Janet B.

AGE:	53
HEIGHT:	5'6"
WEIGHT:	130 lbs
DRESS SIZE:	4
# OF CHILDREN:	3
PROFESSION:	nutritionist, health and fitness expert, author

Janet B.

I have struggled with my weight for years because, quite frankly, I LOVE to eat! In fact, I was almost fired as a flight attendant because at my six-month weigh-in, I had ballooned above my maximum limit! After going on every fad diet on the planet, I finally decided to learn the science behind weight control. What follows is the program that worked for me and continues to work to this day.

I eat small, frequent meals such as breakfast, lunch, and dinner, along with one or two snacks. I eat lots of carbs, but stick to healthy ones such as fruits, vegetables, and whole grains. I also include lean protein and good fats at each meal, eating mostly plant foods with some fish on occasion. I drink low or calorie-free liquids such as coffee and green tea, and I make sure to have a lot of water throughout the day. I rarely eat fried, high-in-fat, or sugary junk foods, but I often treat myself to a small amount of dark chocolate. I also allow myself a nice glass of red wine at dinner.

For exercise, I do up to an hour of daily cardio, and weight train three times a week.

I don't think about my weight much anymore, but make a point to step on a scale every month or so just to make sure I stay on track.

"I often treat myself to a small amount of dark chocolate."

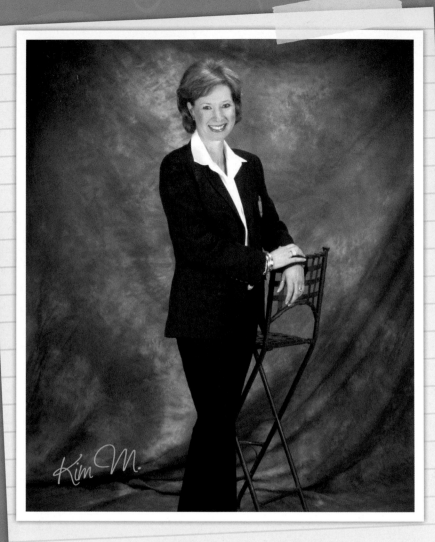

Kim M.

AGE: 53
HEIGHT: 5'6"
WEIGHT: 130 lbs
DRESS SIZE: 4/6
OF CHILDREN: 1
PROFESSION: artist, teacher, inspirational speaker, author

Kim M.

I had struggled with my weight ever since I can remember, but the last three years had been a true battle with the scale! Diet and exercise routines that had worked before weren't working anymore, and I was running out of steam. Then I discovered Weight Watchers. I followed the program and, lo and behold, lost all the weight that I had gained! The points program enabled me to take—and KEEP—the weight off. I now have more energy and my outlook on life has changed for the better. I faithfully keep a food journal, so I can hold myself accountable for everything I put into my mouth. My motto is, "If you bite it, write it!" Also, one of the big "ah-ha!" moments for me was learning about portion sizes.

Today I eat three meals and two snacks such as an apple or a protein smoothie. I enjoy a variety of vegetables such as spaghetti squash, eggplant, and all kinds of salad. I treat myself at restaurants, but won't overeat and often take home half of my dinner for another meal. I avoid fried, sugary, and high-fat foods. I also drink eight glasses of water a day.

My favorite exercises are yoga and walking.

Being able to lose weight and keep it off has led me on an exciting path of self-discovery. As a result, I feel better and have more patience, tolerance, and understanding toward others. Because I finally love myself for who I am, I am in love with life!

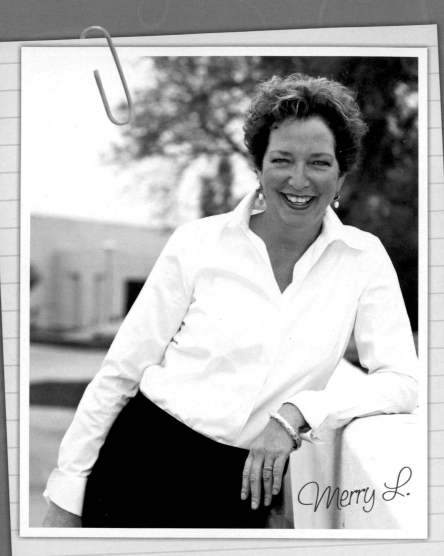

Merry L.

AGE:	54
HEIGHT:	5'7"
WEIGHT:	135 lbs
DRESS SIZE:	6
# OF CHILDREN:	2
PROFESSION:	lifestyle expert, entrepreneur

Merry L.

Several times throughout my adulthood I have gained weight due to overeating. It usually has to do with something specific that's going on at the time. It's an indication that something's eating me, and I use this weight gain as an opportunity to get back on track.

When I'm on target, I eat three meals a day with small snacks in between. If I go for carbs, I eat them for breakfast. I don't buy things like potato chips or popcorn, because they cause me to feel sluggish and moody—which in turn affects those around me. Because I'm on the run a lot, I have to make a special point to find a grocery store so I can pick up a protein bar and some fresh fruit. That way I know my energy and frame of mind will remain positive. While going through menopause, I find it invaluable to supplement with vitamin C, CoQ10, a multivitamin, and potassium.

For exercise, I hike, walk, swim, and do yoga and Zumba®. And to keep it interesting, I love to listen to motivational CDs or tapes while I'm exercising.

Eating well and keeping active is a way of life I've become accustomed to. I also include a mediation practice and recite positive affirmations throughout the day. I don't think about the scale too much. Instead, I consider my energy level, mental clarity, and whether I'm proactively moving toward achieving my goals. If I fit into my clothes, maintain a positive outlook on life, and am pleasant to be around, my weight is barely an issue!

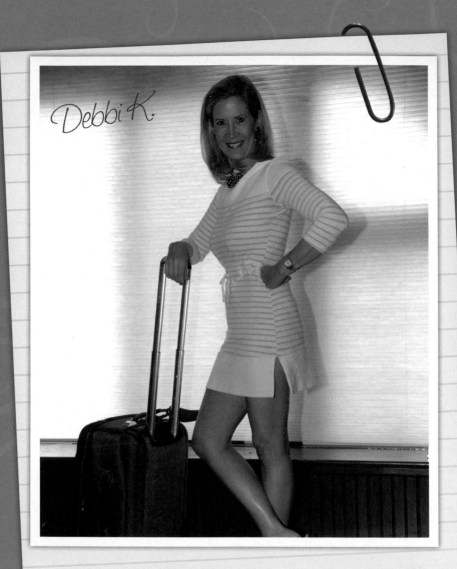

Debbi K.

AGE: 54

HEIGHT: 5'4"

WEIGHT: 109 lbs

DRESS SIZE: 4

PROFESSION: travel writer, marketing consultant, author of The Globetrotter's Get-Gorgeous Guide

Debbi K.

No one loves a meal more than I do! Yet I constantly monitor myself because, to me, no food is worth eating if it's going to put a spare tire around my waist! I have invested in a closet full of lovely clothes and they all fit. I used to be able to stay thin simply by exercising and giving up dessert. Now that I'm older, I count calories to maintain my weight.

I'm a creature of habit. For breakfast, I eat a bowl of Kashi or puffed wheat with skim milk and raisins. For lunch, I make a smoothie with nonfat cottage cheese, pure pumpkin, pumpkin-pie spice, and Splenda—tons of protein! My mid-afternoon snack is fruit or a 90-calorie English muffin with nonfat powdered peanut butter. I'm happiest when I'm munching raisins, chocolate-covered figs, or a handful of cocoa-dusted almonds. For dinner, I eat tons of vegetables, lean protein, and a baked potato topped with no-calorie butter spray. If I'm still hungry, I have a low-fat yogurt or a piece of fruit. I also live on Minute Maid 15-calorie-per-glass lemonade. I practice portion control and make substitutions for things I crave. For example, I love pizza, so I make chicken cacciatore with mushrooms and it almost tastes like pizza, but without the bread! If I'm craving pasta, it's 40-calorie shirataki noodles instead. I avoid fattening cookies, cakes, and pies, and I don't drink alcohol.

I walk three miles daily on the treadmill, perform abdominal and arm exercises every day, and do weights three times a week. I want to be thin—I love being thin—but it is hard work. I always ask myself, "Do I want to eat whatever I want, or do I want to wear whatever I want?" Since I love beautiful clothes, I rarely skip a workout.

Nothing tastes as good as being thin feels. That's my motto, and as long as I keep that in mind, I won't have to spend money on a new wardrobe anytime soon!

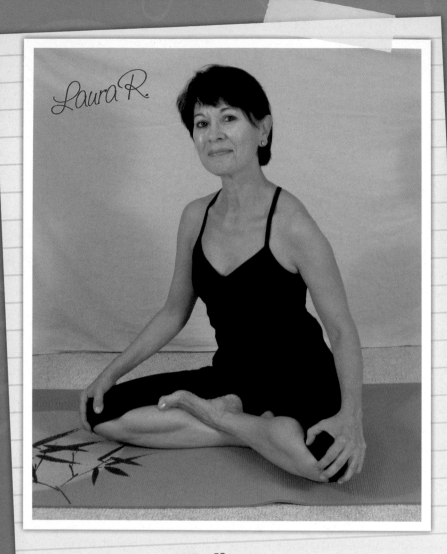

Laura R.

AGE:	55
HEIGHT:	5'2"
WEIGHT:	95 lbs
DRESS SIZE:	0/2
# OF CHILDREN:	2
PROFESSION:	research analyst, inspirational speaker, writer

Laura R.

Although I was a slim child and teenager, I was born uncoordinated, a consummate non-athlete. Since I never made a sports team in high school, I did not exercise and feared turning into a couch potato. However, at age 15 I discovered and taught myself the basics of hatha yoga by reading books and magazines. I did yoga off and on the next few years. When I turned 25, I decided that if I were to stay slim the rest of my life, I'd have to make a permanent commitment to daily aerobic exercise along with yoga. I began with a 10-minute jog and eventually worked up to a 30-minute run. The result was that I ended up with a long, lean, toned look, and I felt wonderful.

Today I avoid red meat, poultry, and dairy products. I eat soy products, veggies, whole grains, and fresh fruit. I indulge in sweets only on occasion. Daily, I drink six to eight cups of water, one cup of coffee with steamed soy milk, one or two cups of herbal tea, and a glass of red wine with dinner. I drink no sodas or fruit juices. I supplement with vitamin E, vitamin D, beta glucan, soy isoflavone, CoQ10, glucosamine, beta carotene, melatonin, calcium, and a multi-mineral tablet.

Four years ago, intent on staying flexible and serene, I put more attention into yoga. I practiced it 25 30 minutes for at least six times a week with great focus. Instead of jogging, I now jump and dance on a mini trampoline for 25 minutes daily and walk two miles round trip from my house to the metro on my go to work

Since following this regime focused on daily exercise and healthy eating, I have maintained my college weight and have a flatter stomach. I look and feel my personal best as a result!

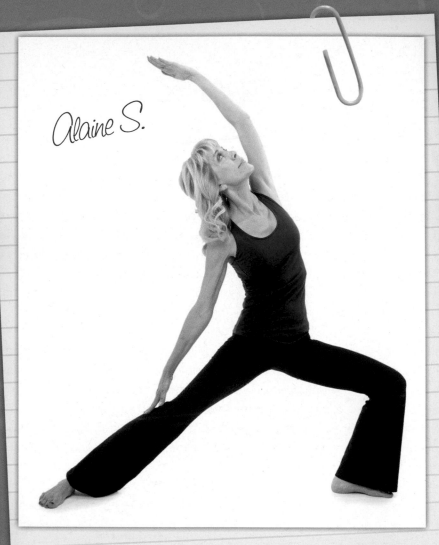

Alaine S.

AGE:	56
HEIGHT:	5'8"
WEIGHT:	113 lbs
DRESS SIZE:	2
PROFESSION:	baker, vegan consultant

Alaine S.

I was slender growing up, but in high school, I put on weight by snacking too much on sweets. When my mother handed me a diet book, I took the hint! I figured out what I could stick to: hot cereal for breakfast, half a cantaloupe with one scoop of ice milk for lunch, and fresh fruit to snack on in the afternoon. For dinner, I ate salad without dressing and a double helping of vegetables—no meat! My rule was no fattening desserts; instead, I had fresh fruit. After a few weeks, I was very pleased with the results. Although I returned to a more typical diet, I ate smaller portions in order to maintain my new weight. I had learned that eating sugary treats was not at all worth being heavier than I wanted to be!

I start my day by drinking water. For breakfast, I always make a smoothie, using an organic, freeze-dried, densely nutritious vegetable, a whole-grain powder mixed with almond milk, and a banana. For dinner, I make vegan dishes such as whole-grain pizza, lasagna, meat-free bean tacos, sweet-potato burritos, or a veggie burger on a sprouted whole-grain bun. I have a large salad sprinkled with granulated kelp and extra-virgin olive oil. Usually I include steamed or roasted vegetables, and an organic, whole-grain combination of millet, brown basmati rice, rye berries, whole-wheat berries, and oat groats. For dessert, I make healthy, nutritious, non-fattening treats that are whole-grain, wheat-free, sugar-free, and fat-free: cakes, pies, tarts, mousses, and cookies. I have been a vegan for 21 years now, and I avoid all animal products. For good health, I don't eat white flour, cane sugar, salt, or processed foods, and I don't drink soda. I eat nothing fried in oil, and only consume oil that naturally occurs in avocados, raw nuts, and whole grains (with the exception of the extra-virgin olive oil on my salad). Before bed I drink more water, totaling eight to ten cups a day.

I exercise every day in dance, strength, and yoga classes, or ride my horse.

Staying active, limber, and strong, as well as living a healthy, vegan lifestyle have kept me feeling and looking great!

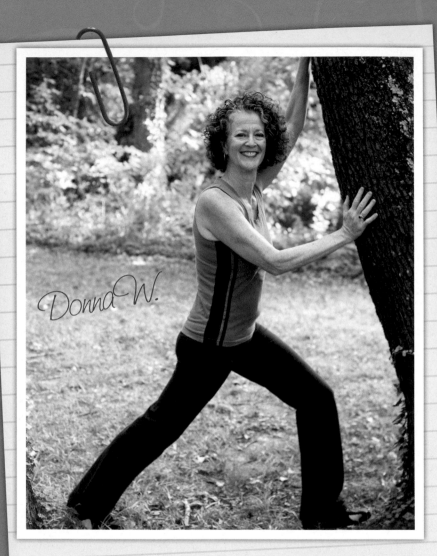

Donna W.

AGE:	56
HEIGHT:	5'5"
WEIGHT:	113 lbs
DRESS SIZE:	2/4
PROFESSION:	massage therapist, health and fitness professional

Donna W.

I never considered myself heavy or overweight. I just had a few pounds settling around the womanly areas: stomach, derriere, and thighs! So I decided to tune in and take cues from my body as to what and when to eat. For example, when having animal protein, I found it digested better with vegetables than with starch, and that bread and cheese made me sleepy. As a result, I began to concentrate on consuming foods that were better for me.

Today I eat a high-protein, low-starch diet. I start the day with fresh vegetable juice, or an almond-milk and whey-protein shake, or eggs and green tea. I buy fresh, high-quality organic vegetables and cook with olive and coconut oil. I avoid cold cuts, soda, wheat, dairy, and anything processed. A typical dinner is lean protein, sweet potato, broccoli, and salad with a glass of wine. For dessert I enjoy fresh fruit and a small piece of dark chocolate. I drink six to eight glasses of alkaline/ionized water a day and supplement with fish oil, calcium, magnesium, vitamin D, vitamin C, liquid trace minerals, and bio-identical hormones.

Twice a week I strength train and on the other days I swim, bike, run, or take an alignment or dance class. I also climb stairs and dance tango.

Increased physical activity paired with a healthy diet has worked well for me. I now know that daily slight errors in judgment can add up and do damage over time. So, I have become conscious to make mindful choices, and as a result, I am now at my ideal weight. It's hard work, but I don't care to risk the alternative!

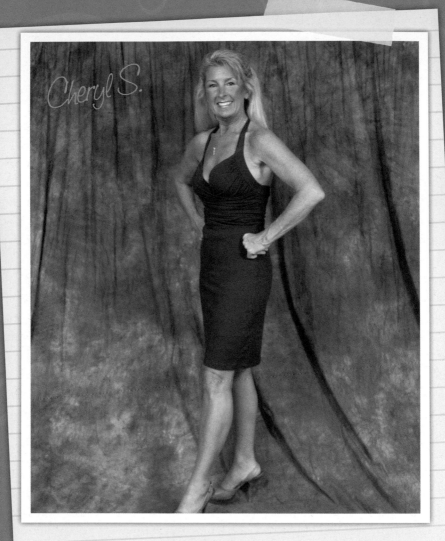

Cheryl S.

AGE: 56

HEIGHT: 5'4"

WEIGHT: 120 lbs

DRESS SIZE: 2/4

OF CHILDREN: 2

PROFESSION: certified hypnotherapist, inspirational speaker

Cheryl S.

When I reached my thirties, I found myself struggling with weight gain. That wasn't such a surprise, as my nutrition was poor and I was inactive. Yet I was always on a diet, which was almost always closely followed by feelings of frustration and failure! Then someone recommended hypnosis. I was at the end of my rope. I figured, what did I have to lose? I wanted it to work, so I was disappointed that nothing seemed to happen. However, over the next few weeks, I seemed to lose that familiar craving for junk food. Instead, I found myself wanting eggs for breakfast and salad for lunch, and I enjoyed the healthier foods so much more!

Today I no longer have an appetite for heavy, greasy, high-calorie foods. I don't care for sweets or soda, and I don't feel the need to eat between meals. What I do have is a desire to consume nutritious, low-calorie meals, and I am motivated to exercise regularly.

For exercise, I go to the gym three times a week. I take an aerobics class or use the stair stepper, and I truly enjoy the physical activity!

I continue to reinforce my good habits by listening to hypnosis CDs, and the mental battles, diets, and worries are now gone! I also experience more relaxation, stress reduction, and deeper sleep. I feel happy, healthy, and more motivated to exercise as well. I eat what I like (which is good, nutritious foods) and have no desire to overeat. I truly am grateful to have found the miracle of hypnosis!

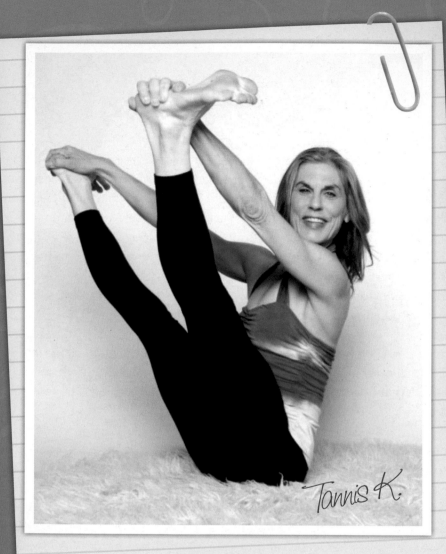

Tannis K.

AGE:	56
HEIGHT:	5'5"
WEIGHT:	114 lbs
DRESS SIZE:	2/4
PROFESSION:	Pilates instructor, owner of a mind-body travel program

Tannis K.

G rowing up, I had the body of a ballerina. When the hormones hit, the curves came, and I struggled to stay thin. In my 20's I gained even more weight, and even though I was teaching aerobics and dieting, the scale wasn't budging! Finally, determined to lose some weight, I lived on cabbage soup and steamed veggies. Once my metabolism stabilized, I lost weight and it stayed off.

Today I aim for a balanced diet. For breakfast, I have oatmeal with milk or eggs and toast. I eat mini-meals such as fruit, cottage cheese, yogurt, a slice of cheese, or some chicken. And when I crave salt, I grab a handful of nuts or a few tortilla chips. I drink a lot of fluids, such as protein shakes, juice, water, tea, and warm-you-up soups in the winter. Chicken or fish—cooked in olive oil, garlic, and spices—along with steamed veggies or salad with a side of dressing, keep the taste buds happy for dinner. I avoid all processed and artificial substances and I never drink soda.

I exercise daily by doing either Pilates or GYROTONIC® (an exercise similar to yoga), and opt for stairs over elevators.

In addition to a sensible diet and moderate exercise, traveling, learning, and treating myself to the occasional new outfit that shows off my unique beauty are the ways I stay healthy and thin.

"Today I aim for a balanced diet."

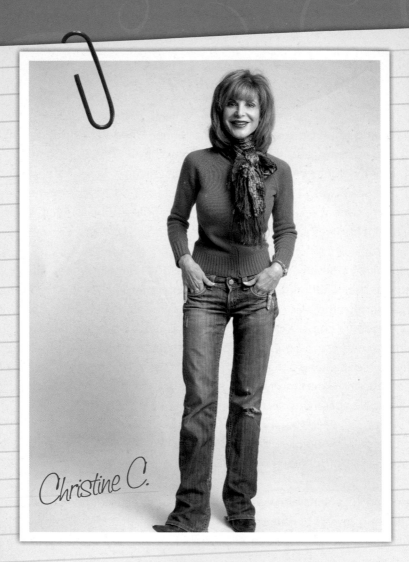

Christine C.

AGE:	56
HEIGHT:	5'6"
WEIGHT:	108 lbs
DRESS SIZE:	0
# OF CHILDREN:	2
PROFESSION:	author, professional speaker, business owner

Christine C.

Although I always ate what I wanted and didn't gain a pound, there is a reason for that. It's called exercise! In my youth, I loved to swim, walk, run, and hike. However, after college I moved to a colder climate and couldn't figure out the best way to exercise with all that snow on the ground! As a result, I gained a few pounds, which I didn't enjoy. There have also been times when I was a bit heavier—following the birth of my two sons, for example. Then there were times when I got too thin—when I suffered through a bout with breast cancer and two divorces. So I went back to a series of calisthenics and free weights I learned in high school and that did the trick. Within a few short months, the pounds were gone or the muscle mass was built again.

Today I eat a diet of lean protein, vegetables, salads, and multi-grain breads. I also enjoy a daily glass of wine and a handful of chocolate. In addition, I take a multivitamin and a supplement called Protandim for free radical and antioxidant protection.

For exercise, I walk four miles a day with my Siberian Husky, golf a few times a week—walking the course rather than riding a cart—and still do calisthenics

I take a holistic view of my health, crediting a fabulous family, fantastic friends, rewarding work, and a lot of laughter for my success!

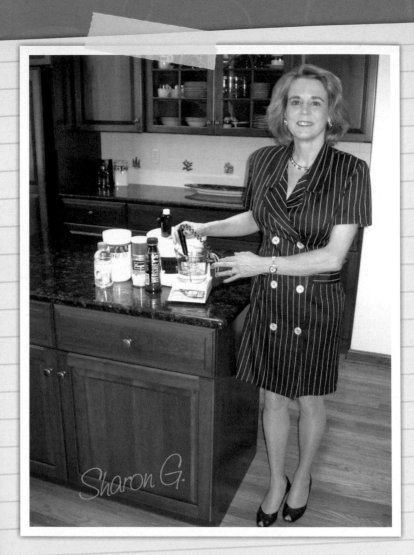

Sharon G.

AGE: 57

HEIGHT: 5'3"

WEIGHT: 105 lbs

DRESS SIZE: 4

 # OF CHILDREN: 3

PROFESSION: author, food scientist

Sharon G.

I grew up on a farm. We worked hard, played hard, and ate hearty. I devoured sour-cream cakes and I never gained a pound. However, when I went to college, I ate heavy dorm food (and more than enjoyed the occasional beer) and thus began my lifelong battle of the bulge. Gradually I quit eating desserts, learned to drink tea in lieu of soda, and stayed active daily. If my weight crept up on vacation or holidays, I cut back on sweets and exercised more until I was back on target. I became fascinated with nutrition, and in the process of getting educated, interviewed and consulted with hundreds of food industry experts. Here is what I learned to do to maintain a healthy and balanced body:

- I jump-start my metabolism by eating breakfast, such as Quaker Weight Control Oatmeal with milk, fruit, and whey protein within 30 minutes of waking.
- I build my diet around a variety of colorful, nutrient-dense foods.
- I practice portion control by eating three sensible meals and several snacks.
- I eat homegrown vegetables (a great source of fiber) and use fresh herbs to season my food.
- I have three servings of dairy, which provide quality protein, calcium, and vitamin D.
- I rarely and sparingly indulge in sweets.
- I exercise daily, enjoying sports such as biking, hiking, aerobics, and resistance exercises. I also like home videos such as Kathy Smith's *Lift Weights to Lose Weight*.

My motto is: The day you stop fighting the battle of the bulge is the day you lose. Maintaining my weight over the years has been a daily regimen of small choices. I take the stairs—not the elevator. I eat the apple—not the pie. And as a result, deciding to eat healthier and exercise more has become an effortless habit over time.

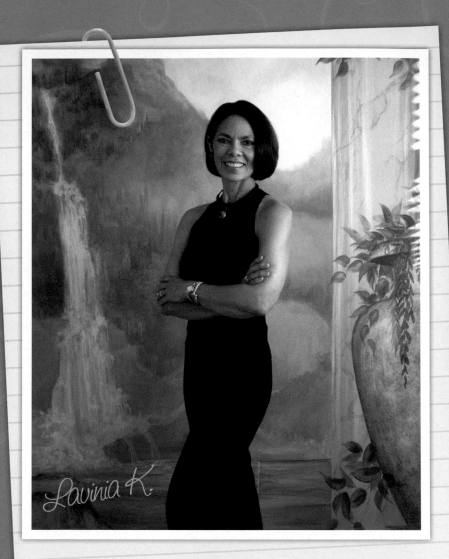

Lavinia K.

AGE: 57

HEIGHT: 5'4"

WEIGHT: 120 lbs

DRESS SIZE: 4

PROFESSION: clinical psychologist

Lavinia K.

Growing up, I didn't like exercise of any kind. To add insult to injury, I was fed a high-fat diet of white rice and beans, fried foods, and little greenery. As a result, I was not fit or healthy. In graduate school I began doing research on obesity and later worked with eating disorders. Through my studies I learned strategies that really helped with losing weight and keeping it off. Ultimately, this effort led to writing a book on the psychology of weight management.

Today I eat four to five times a day, concentrating on a high-complexity-carb, low-fat diet. I consume mostly healthy, nutritious foods with lots of veggies, fruit ,and whole grains, and keep bad fats, sweets, and processed foods to a minimum. I take a casual approach to portion control by eating from smaller plates. This works just fine, as long as I take my time! I also make sure to have a large glass of water with each meal. I supplement with a multivitamin, probiotics, omega-3, calcium, vitamin D3, and glucosamine.

I walk for an hour a day and incorporate muscle-resistance training three times per week.

My philosophy is basically that the more rigid your approach is to weight and fitness, the less successful you will be. Making sure that things are flexible, having patience, and taking approaches that can be followed for a lifetime are the basics of success with weight management and health.

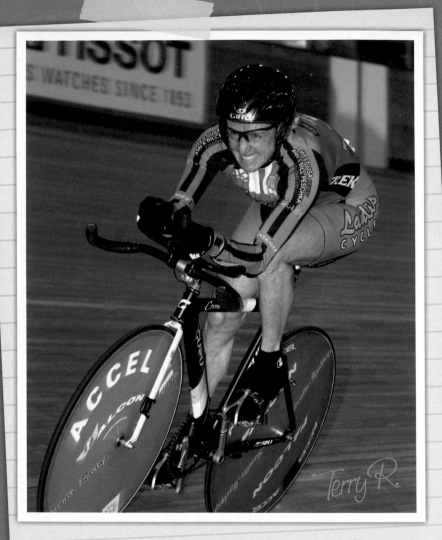

AGE:	58
HEIGHT:	5'5"
WEIGHT:	132 lbs
DRESS SIZE:	4/6
# OF CHILDREN:	2
PROFESSION:	registered kinesiotherapist

Terry R.

In high school and beyond, I stayed active as a runner, skier, tennis player, and triathlete turned cyclist. When competitively bike racing, I avoided sweets and alcohol and exercised 20 hours a week. Because of the intensity of my training, I ate huge volumes of food five to six times a day to keep my fuel source up, replenish my muscle mass, and give me the energy needed to perform at my best. However, when I hit my fifth decade and underwent a neck fusion operation, I started experiencing a middle-age frump. I cut out starchy bread, pasta, and sugary sweets. I bumped up my intensity and duration on the bike, and was able to return to a comfortable weight within a few short months.

Today, breakfast consists of eggs, flourless toast, peanut butter, banana, and tea. Lunch is a protein sandwich with lots of veggies and fruit for dessert. For dinner, I stick to protein and salad, or potato and vegetable, and a glass of wine.

My exercise routine now is biking ten hours a week to maintain my current weight. If work and life get in the way, I gain weight in a heartbeat.

I do enjoy splurging on the "forbidden foods," but proper nutrition and exercise—coupled with high-intensity efforts to bump up my heart rate—do the trick for me!

"I started experiencing a middle-age frump."

"Few people know how to take a walk.
The qualifications are endurance,
plain clothes, old shoes, an eye for nature,
good humor, vast curiosity, good speech,
good silence, and nothing too much."

~Ralph Waldo Emerson

The
60's

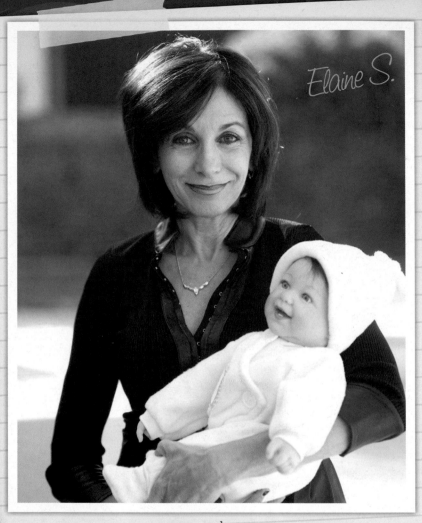

Elaine S.

AGE:	ageless
HEIGHT:	5'2"
WEIGHT:	105
DRESS SIZE:	2
# OF CHILDREN:	1
PROFESSION:	author, psychologist, speaker, trainer, parent educator, speech-language pathologist

Elaine S.

When I was in my 20's, friends would indulge in hot dogs, pizza and soft drinks, while I would eat from a baggie of raisins and nuts, drink water, and be perfectly content. I viewed my body as a temple and lived with the saying, "You are what you eat and think." I realized I could fill my body with junk and carry around extra baggage, or keep myself trim and healthy. I also did yoga and danced.

What do I eat today? Poultry, fish, grains, fruits, vegetables, and nuts. I took an allergy test and found that I was both lactose- and wheat-intolerant. I am now on a gluten-free, wheat-free, sodium-free, and lactose-free diet. As a result of eliminating these substances, my stomach is no longer bloated and I have a lot more energy! I avoid eating processed foods, red meat, and sugar, and drink plenty of water (and tea) throughout the day. I take supplements by opening the capsules and stirring their contents into sugar-free cinnamon applesauce for quick absorption.

For exercise, I start each day by stretching in an effort to stay limber and strong. I do cardio, lift weights, and work with a personal trainer once a week as well.

I meditate twice a day, visualizing myself at my perfect weight, knowing that whatever I eat will nourish me and the rest will leave my body. I keep myself balanced with healthy food, exercise, meditation, a loving family, great friends, and by performing good deeds daily. Waking up with a gratitude attitude recharges me daily.

Note: The baby in the photo is my lifelike doll, on whom I demonstrate baby massage strokes for caregivers, parents, and professionals. Joy is easy to carry, but there are real grandchildren in my future. Therefore, I want to stay fit so as to be able to carry them around with ease when the time comes!

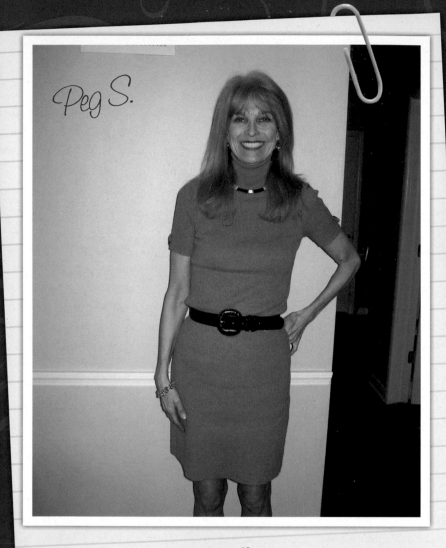

Peg S.

AGE:	60
HEIGHT:	5'8"
WEIGHT:	116 lbs
DRESS SIZE:	0/2
# OF CHILDREN:	1
PROFESSION:	author

Peg S.

I was quite slight growing up. But once my metabolism changed, I noticed that what I usually ate was now putting on the pounds! I began daily aerobics and paid more attention to what I was eating. But after giving birth, I just couldn't shake the post-pregnancy pounds—at least with whatever I was doing at the time! A few years later I became so uncomfortable that I finally decided to learn what it took to maintain a healthy weight once and for all.

Today breakfast is eggs or a mixture of strawberries, blueberries, and bananas. Lunch is cottage cheese, cherry tomatoes, and an apple. For a snack, I have a handful of plain, raw almonds. Dinner is grilled chicken and a vegetable such as broccoli, asparagus, peppers, or a salad with homemade dressing. I stay away from prepared or packaged foods containing sodium, gluten, or fat. I drink plenty of water throughout the day, and enjoy a glass of wine with dinner. I take supplements such as vitamin C, vitamin D, vitamin E, calcium, flax seed oil, and MSM for joint health as well.

My exercise regimen is walking briskly two to four miles every day. Six months after I started walking, I had to have all of my skirts altered—no more hips! In an effort to avoid a plateau, I also work out on the Total Gym® followed by an ab roller for toning.

In this way, I have maintained the same weight for the last decade. If my clothes start feeling snug, I just go a couple of days without bread, pasta, or rice and see an almost immediate change in my waistline. Staying active is the true fountain of youth and the secret to my ability to remain slim.

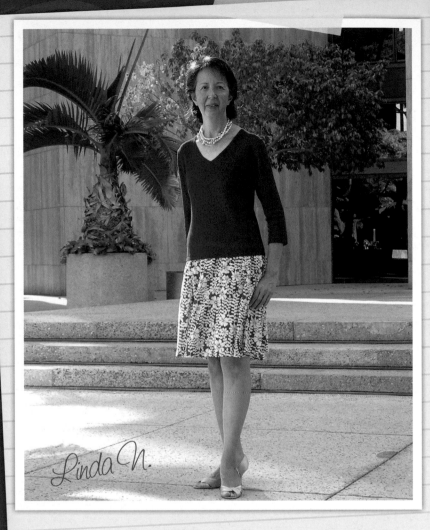

Linda N.

AGE:	60
HEIGHT:	5'7"
WEIGHT:	115 lbs
DRESS SIZE:	4
PROFESSION:	inventor, company founder

Linda N.

I am thin, it's true. Yet I gained a bit of weight in college when I was not paying much attention to what I was putting into my body.

Today my routine is to have a light breakfast of cereal and fresh fruit. Lunch is a chicken or tuna sandwich with lettuce and tomatoes or a selection of sushi. For dinner, I have chicken or fish and green-leaf lettuce salad with cucumber, spinach, carrots, and tomatoes. I also include healthy carbs such as brown rice, whole-wheat pasta, and whole-grain breads. I stay away from candy, cake, pie, and sweets. I drink three to four glasses of water per day, and take a multivitamin and some additional D-3 to supplement my diet.

In addition to walking my dogs twice a day, I work out on a Pilates machine 40–60 minutes every other day.

My philosophy is that I eat to live. In this way I am able to maintain a slender frame, which makes me feel energetic, happy, and peaceful within. I am not preoccupied with my weight, but being slim just feels right for me.

"My philosophy is that I eat to live"

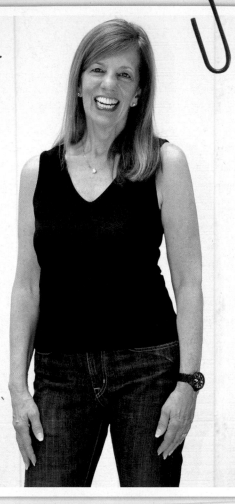

Sharon O.

AGE:	60
HEIGHT:	5'4"
WEIGHT:	122 lbs
DRESS SIZE:	6
# OF CHILDREN:	1
PROFESSION:	marriage and family therapist, author

Sharon O.

I grew up in an era when girls didn't play sports, and honestly, I didn't want to sweat! After my son was born in my mid-30's, I was determined to shed any uncomfortable excess weight, so I joined a gym and started lifting weights. I also invested in a NordicTrack®, and over time, discovered that I loved running, hiking, and all things outdoors!

Today I eat two meals a day with small snacks in between. Breakfast is yogurt, fresh fruit, eggs, or oatmeal. I snack on raw almonds, protein bars, chickpeas, pickles, and dried fruit. Dinner is chicken, salmon, turkey meatloaf, vegetables, salad, and a glass of wine. If I get hungry before bed, I have hummus or salsa with low-fat crackers, baby carrots, or some cereal. Here are some additional behaviors that have made a positive difference in maintaining my weight:

- I weigh myself daily with a scale that includes a fat monitor.
- I have hot water with lemon juice and a few shakes of Cayenne pepper every morning.
- I add cranberry juice to water and drink four to five glasses a day.

- I relax and enjoy my meals, eat very slowly and make sure to stop before I'm full.
- I choose stairs over elevators when possible.
- I avoid fried and fast foods, sugar, fat, and salt, opting for olive oil, sea salt, low-fat dairy, and whole wheat over anything white.
- During the holidays, I make a big pot of vegetable soup and fill up between special meals and treats.
- When at a restaurant, I share meals or take home half in a doggie bag.
- I drink a cup of tea before dinner.
- I try my best to get a minimum of seven hours of sleep each night.
- If I have a splurge during the week, I carry on as usual.

For exercise, I enjoy yoga, lifting weights, and working out on a treadmill for 30–60 minutes, six days a week.

Learning how to sweat—and loving it—has enabled me to maintain a healthy, slender body. I have come to appreciate the constant, little decisions that have become second nature to me. For someone who loves to eat, exercise has made all the difference in my weight year in and year out.

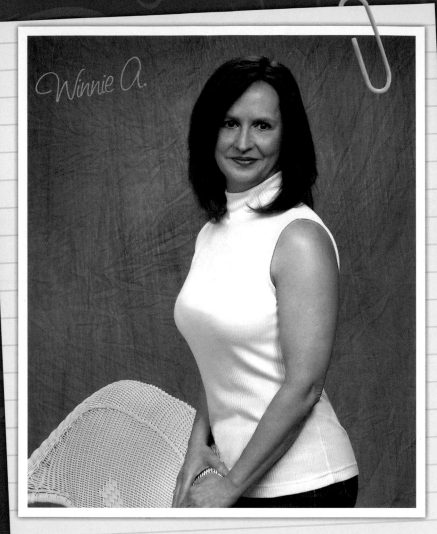

Winnie A.

AGE: 60

HEIGHT: 5'2"

WEIGHT: 115 lbs

DRESS SIZE: 6

PROFESSION: marketing strategist

Winnie A.

E ven though I was thin as a child, after I grew up and started working, life became sedentary. To my dismay I found myself living life as a pleasantly plump adult. One day I saw Richard Simons on a talk show. He stuck his fist in a bowl overflowing with chicken fat, explaining that his hand represented human organs surrounded by lard. If this didn't motivate me, I don't know what did! It took me several months, but I eventually lost the weight through exercise, portion control, and making smarter choices—no more muffin-like treats for breakfast!

Today I eat a small, healthy breakfast followed by a moderate-sized lunch and a light dinner. I snack on fruit, low-fat cheese, and/or nuts during the day, avoiding sugar and processed foods. If I crave a treat such as ice cream I'll indulge, but I control the portion by choosing a child's size cone or a popsicle. I drink a lot of water and tea and supplement with a daily multivitamin.

I work out daily or every other day. I work out with home video programs, favoring those that include simple moves that leverage body weight. As a result, I've learned that building muscle helps burn fat.

I weigh myself each morning and plan my meals in advance to keep myself on track. I've found that chewing gum during stressful times helps manage mindless eating. Having been on both sides of the fence, I can say that the things that I do to remain thin are worth every sacrifice. Being healthy and slim are of prime importance to me, and no food or lack of focus would be worth gaining again!

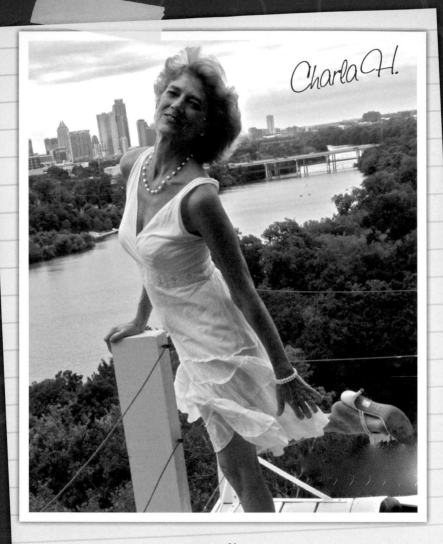

Charla H.

AGE:	61
HEIGHT:	5'7"
WEIGHT:	124
DRESS SIZE:	4
# OF CHILDREN:	1
PROFESSION:	author, speaker, couples retreat leader

Charla H.

I maintained a healthy weight up to about the age of 40. At that point I was shocked to see the number on the scale go up and up, so I decided to take action before it got any worse. I began reducing my portions and eating mindfully by chewing food better and putting my fork down between bites. To quote my acupuncturist, "Chew your drink and drink your food." I also cut out dairy and dessert. In addition, I got into the habit of taking food home in a doggie bag when eating out, rather than finishing my plate.

Today I read labels before purchasing food. I avoid boxed and processed items containing sugar and preservatives. I avoid wheat because I find it disrupts my digestion, but I do add brown rice, oat groats, millet, and a gaggle of greens each day to my meals. I pay attention to food combinations and avoid meat, carbs, and dairy in the same meal. For sweeteners I use agave, which has a low-glycemic index. I drink six to eight glasses of water per day and do not eat after 7 p.m. I cut out hydrogenated fats and replaced them with healthful ones such as flaxseed and fish oil. I also take a probiotic and digestive enzyme, and each spring I do a cleanse.

My exercise routine consists of 30 minutes of yoga followed by a 20-minute walk each day. I go to bed early and get up early. The Chinese proverb states, "One hour of sleep before midnight is worth two after." According to ancient Chinese medicine, organs rejuvenate during the night and the sun's light has a strong effect on healing rhythms.

These lifestyle and diet changes have made me feel lighter on my feet, more energetic, and more interested in life than ever before!

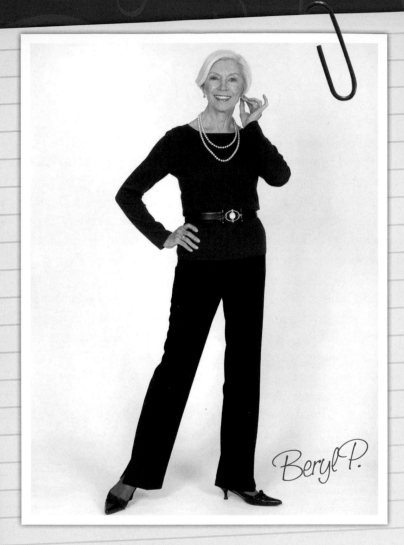

Beryl P.

AGE: 69
HEIGHT: 5'7"
WEIGHT: 115 lbs
DRESS SIZE: 4/6
PROFESSION: certified image consultant

Beryl P.

My weight has remained stable for over forty years, but that was not always the case. I grew up on a cattle ranch where we had fresh vegetables and hearty meals of fried meat, salad, vegetables, potatoes, and gravy. There were cookies in the jar and cakes or pies for dessert every day. You could say I had an ample figure! After graduating, I became curious about nutrition, so I began to check ingredients on labeled grocery items. "If you can't pronounce it, don't eat it" became my guide. This eliminated junk and processed foods from my diet, and within a few months I began to see a slimmer me. I was most delighted to discover I actually had a shape!

For breakfast, I have a protein-powder shake with filtered water, ice, a banana, and frozen berries. When I start the day with protein, my blood sugar—which causes hunger—doesn't drop as much during the day. My lunch is soup and/or salad and a handful of raw almonds for an afternoon snack. For dinner, I have a lean meat such as fish or chicken, steamed vegetables, and salad followed by a glass of wine. If have a yearning for a starchy potato, bread, or dessert, I will eat a small portion or share a serving with a friend. I have no desire for fried foods or anything laden with chemicals. I drink eight glasses of water per day, and supplement with a doctor-recommended multivitamin.

For exercise, I take a brisk walk for at least 30 minutes five or six times a week.

There have been some adjustments and modifications over the years, but my diet remains clean and I continue to make physical activity a priority. My aunt Jane followed a healthy lifestyle and was still designing her own clothes and driving to and from her dressmaker at the age of 95. I want to be just like Aunt Jane!

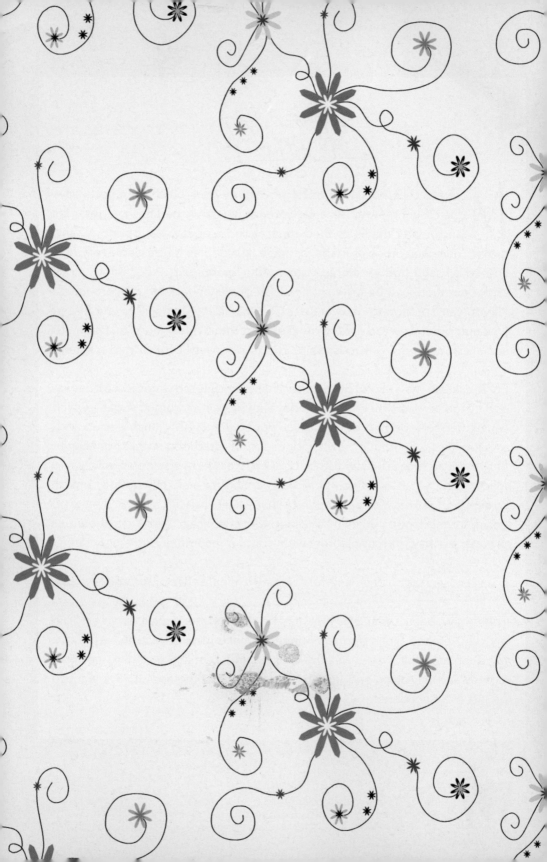

Conclusion

What I came to realize was that although there are some woman who are and have always been thin, many rely on exercise and healthy eating habits to maintain their weight. Even the women who said things like, "I've been thin my entire life. I'm just lucky, I guess," upon further investigation, came to find that they eat small meals throughout the day, avoid processed foods and sugar like the plague, rarely drink soda or eat after 8 p.m., drink lots of water, take nutritional supplements, do yoga, go to the gym, and do weight-bearing exercises come hell or high water because having a healthy body is a priority to them. Now, that sounds like discipline to me! And whatever their disciplines or habits are, it has become a way of life.

As the stories poured in, I slowly got both the information and inspiration I needed to move forward toward my own weight-loss goals. I realized that the problem was not nearly as simple as what I was putting in my mouth. Rather, the solutions ultimately hinged on just how much and when, nutritional supplementation, learning how to counteract insurmountable cravings, and the importance of weight-bearing exercises.

During this time, I was introduced to three things. First, I was introduced to a five-day plan that reset my blood sugar and insulin regulation. As a result, I was not as hungry, ate less, and made healthier choices. Second, I started taking an antioxidant blend that gave my body the energy I hadn't had in nearly a decade. And third, I began working out at home with a video series based on exercising different muscles daily, and started weight-bearing exercises. So between beating the formerly impossible cravings, having the energy for daily exercise, and enlisting an online coach who held me accountable to my workouts, I decided to commit to succeed in losing weight and keeping it off for good! My goal was to be able to contribute a story to this book. I prayed for the strength to remain disciplined. I prayed for health and for my body to change shape. And I purposely reserved a place for myself, because I was visualizing success.

I am proud to say that I have claimed a spot in *Is She Naturally Thin or Disciplined?* And I am more empowered and successful than the thought of weight loss itself, because I feel better than ever before, understand what mistakes I was making, and know what I am now doing correctly. I am exercising regularly with weights as well as putting good things into my body at the correct intervals throughout the day, and taking proper nutrients to battle those crazy cravings!

Discipline is not an easy road, far from it. But is it worth it? I know that it is! I want to thank every woman in this book for helping to educate us about the importance of proper nutrition and supplementation, and for inspiring us to incorporate exercise into our lives as a lifestyle choice. And just as I suspected, over time, these disciplines have begun to feel natural to me as well.

My wish is that those who are struggling, discouraged, and looking for answers, will receive the same inspiration and education I did from these honest, forthright, heartfelt, and caring stories. Each contributor has opened up with a very detailed account as to how she maintains her beautiful frame in order to help us all, and for that I am eternally grateful!

So, as for the query in the title of this book, I have found my answer. The answer is quite clear—it's discipline! And that discipline eventually turns into a natural way of life. Kudos and appreciation to this hard-working and focused group of ladies!

To quote the BeachBody slogan, "Decide. Commit. Succeed!®"

Sally Shields

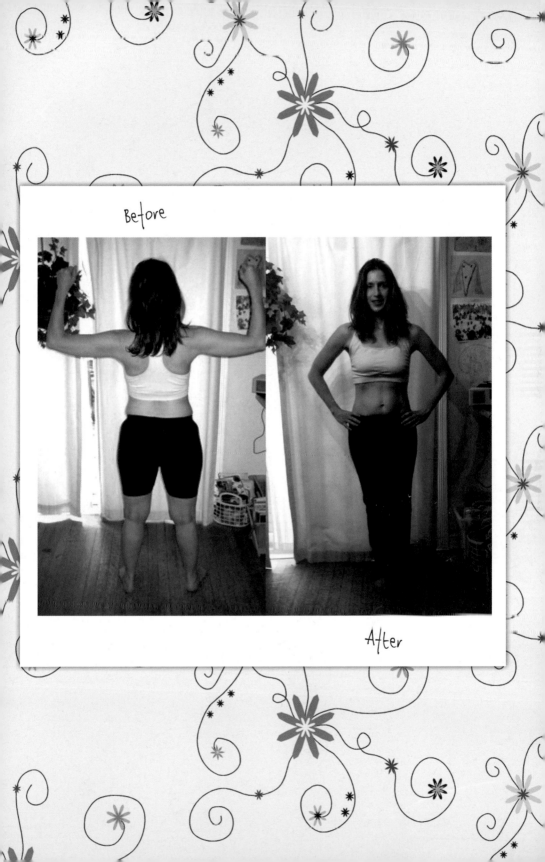

Before

After

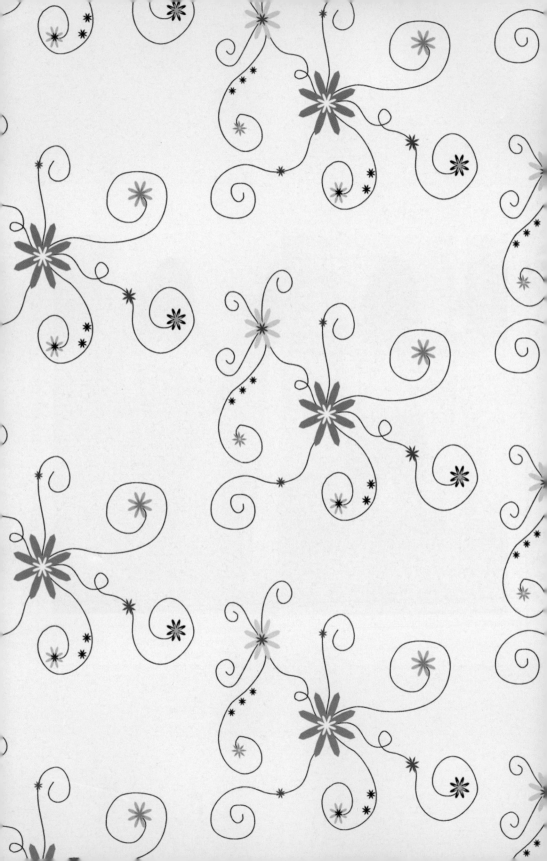

Acknowledgements

A Very Special Thanks to:

Jamie Gough, Kent Gustavson, Carolyn Sheltraw, Kristina Tosic, Debbi Kickham, David Kimelman, Lara Palombi, Phil and Lorenzo, Audrey Welber, Kathleen Pleasants, Donna Marie Merritt, Ashley Van Winkle, Camila Tessler, Cara Selick, Elizabeth Fink, Janice Paterson, Laura Daill, Margaret Smith, Laura Strickland, Ronnie Horowitz and, of course, all the incredible contributors within these pages!

In addition, a VERY EXTRA special thanks to Victoria Dunckley, Suzy Stauffer and Tony Horton, without whom I never would have been able to include myself in this book.

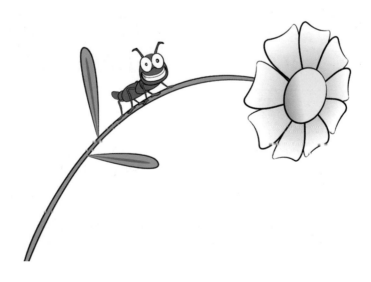

My ♥ Belongs to

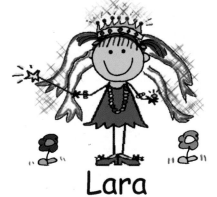

Lara

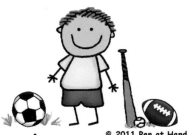

© 2011 Pen at Hand, Inc.

Lorenzo

About the Author

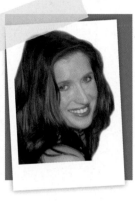

Sally Shields is a musician and composer, and now, a dedicated fitness enthusiast. After having kids, she could no longer travel the world or stay out late hanging out at jazz clubs while simultaneously getting up at the break-of dawn and being mom all day—so she turned to writing. Her first book, *The Daughter-in-Law Rules: 101 Surefire Ways to Make Friends with Your Mother-in-Law* was inspired by tricky nuances that arose with her very own mother-in-law. The book ended up featured in many media outlets, and as a result became a #1 Amazon.com bestseller. Then, in an effort to assist other self-published authors on a tight budget, she penned *Publicity Secrets Revealed: What Every PR Firm Doesn't Want You to Know*. Her third book, *The Collaborator Rules: 101 Surefire Ways to Stay Friends with Your Co-Author* was born out of a subsequent and less-than-stellar collaborative experience, and serves to educate those who are ruminating about the joys of creative-partnerships. She is now happily co-editor of The Speaker Anthology series, which was designed to provide speakers with a book of their very own to sell at their events around the globe.

Through it all, Sally's very own her battle-of-the-bulge had her looking at skinny women everywhere, and wondering how exactly they maintained their trim and healthy frames. So she decided to ask them. A lot of them. 101 of them. Her successful weight-loss journey led to a passion for wanting to share the benefit of her experience with others, and that is what led her to pen, *Is She Naturally Thin? Or Disciplined? Insider Secrets of the Sexy and Slim!* Living in NYC, Sally continues to write, compose and perform, but mostly stays local so she can always be home to cuddle her kids. For more info, please visit www.sallyshields.com.

Contributors

Alaine Shrewsbury is a healthy, whole-grain, vegan baker who also teaches people how to clean up their diets so they feel stronger. www.greenheartbakery.com

Alexis Buntin is the brand manager for Reserveage Organics, a leading health supplement company. www.reserveage. com (Photo credit: Alexander Davidowski of Mirador Studios)

Alicia Dunams is a speaker, coach, and author. www.goaldigger.com and www. aliciadunams.com

Angel Tuccy is the host of a daily radio show and bestselling author. She is also founder of Experience Pros University and she sits on the Board of Directors for the Chamber of Commerce of Highlands Ranch. www. ExperiencePros.com

Angela Manzanares is the founder of fit-losophy and creator of fitbook™, a revolutionary line of fitness plus nutrition journals that are redefining how people reach their fitness goals. www.getfitbook.com

Angela Suthrave is a registered dietician and is active as a counselor, writer, and speaker. www.delightfulnutrition.com

Antoinette Miller is a contributing writer for African American Golfer's Digest, model, and up-and coming author. She is the Editor-in-Chief of online magazine FBENOW for young entrepreneurs. www.fbenow.com

Becky Fox is owner of a fitness and weight-loss company designed to help women drop unwanted body fat and get in the best shape ever! www.foxfitness.com (Photo credit: H.E. Images)

Beryl Pleasants is a certified image consultant who guides each client to discover a true identity deep down inside. Combined with physical attributes, each individual will confidently project his/her signature style or brand. www.stylewithaplomb.com

Brett Blumenthal combined her passion for wellness and her seasoned experience in consulting to establish a company to help people find health easily, naturally, and sustainably. www.sheerbalance.com and www. thehealthyroadwarrior.com

Candy Keane is a costume designer and owner of a costume boutique and Web site for women who love costumes and dressing up for Halloween, theme parties, club nights, or even a sexy night in. www. ThreeMusesClothing.com (Photo credit: Vincent Pierce)

Chantaye McLaughlin is CEO of Urban Integrity, a business consulting company, a private lender, humanitarian, entrepreneur and author. www.Chantaye.org and www. iamchantaye.wordpress.com

Charla Hathaway, sex and intimacy coach and author, makes good lovers great, and satisfied couples sublime! She speaks on Selling to Your Most Important Client—Your Lover, and How to Close the Sale in the Bedroom. www.bodyjoy.org

Charly Emery is a personal strategist. With an effective alternative to traditional coaching/therapy that saves you valuable time and money, she is quickly becoming the face of a newer, swifter, and more savvy self-help model. www.CharlySense.com

Cheryl Savage is a mental health specialist and certified hypnotherapist who has exceptional success with her clients to help them live happier, healthier lives more abundantly. *www.TheHypnosisQueen.com*

Christina Smith is a pilot, philanthropist, and personal finance expert, whose passion is helping people realize their financial goals. She is also the creator of the stepUP movement which highlights everyday heroes in the community. *www.highroadinvestments.com*

Christine Binnendyk is an author and trainer who teaches Pilates at the Nike World Headquarters in Portland, OR. *www.Ageless-Pilates.com*

Christine Clifford is an award-winning speaker, bestselling author, and producer of a beautiful DVD entitled *One Move at a Time! Exercise for Women Recovering from Breast Cancer Surgery*. Don't forget to laugh!™ *www.ChristineClifford.com* and *www.CancerClub.com*

Colleen Riddle is a certified pre/postnatal exercise specialist and creator of the New Mommy Makeover postnatal weight-loss system. She also owns Elite Physique Personal Training, LLC. *www.NewMommyMakeover.com* and *www.ElitePhysiquePT.com*

Dawn McIntyre is a spiritual, intuitive, bestselling author and expert in leading men and women into higher states of expansion and beauty consciousness. *www.boldlybeautiful.com*

Debbi Kickham is a travel writer and marketing consultant who specializes in representing plastic surgeons, cosmetic dentists, hair salons, and spas. Debbi is also the author of the *The Globetrotter's Get-Gorgeous Guide*, the world's first diet and beauty book for traveling women. *www.MarketingAuthor.com* and *www.Gorgeousglobetrotter.com*

Debi Silber is a registered dietitian, personal trainer, whole health coach, speaker, and author. Debi teaches women how to become their personal and professional best. *www.TheMojoCoach.com*

Deborah Poland is the creator of exclusive, handmade designs of chic sport jewelry that will take you wherever you want to go in style. *www.SportyChicDesigns.com*

DeeAnn Donovan is an international fitness model, radio and television personality, former Mrs. New York International™, personal trainer, health and nutrition advocate, life coach, figure competitor, and mom of three. *www.DeeAnnsDayDreamBeliever.com*

Diana Ma has a background in management and marketing. A wedding planner extraordinaire, her gifts include organizing, coordinating, and making all things pretty. *dianamaweddings.com* (Photo credit: Rodeo Photography)

Doll Avant is a singer/songwriter/actress/musician. *www.dollavant.com*

Donna Lewczuk is a mortgage broker and mother of three. *www.DonnasMortgages.com*

Donna Sozio is a dating expert, author, and publishing consultant. Her books *Never Trust a Man in Alligator Loafers* and *The Man Whisperer* have been featured on *Tyra Banks, The Early Show*, Match.com, Yahoo! Personals, and more. *www.donnasozio.com*

Dr. Donna Thomas-Rodgers has established a company focused on world class leadership. Her mission is to lead with style, encouraging clients to present their best in all facets of their professional and personal development. *www.thepowerstarters.com*

Donna Waks is a certified massage and craniosacral therapist, certified movement analyst, and Yamuna® body rolling practitioner. She offers a multi-modal approach to wellness, living fully, and aging gracefully. *www.fluidbody-fluidmovement.com*

Dr. Elaine Schneider is an expert in the field of verbal and nonverbal communication. Award-winning speech-language pathologist, she is a sought-after public speaker and radio show personality. She is also the author of *Massaging Your Baby: The Joy of Touch Time*, subtitled *Effective Techniques for a Happier, Healthier, More Relaxed Child & Parent*. www.touchtimeinternational.com

Dr. Elizabeth Lambaer is a gifted inspirational speaker, talk show host, interviewer, and Vitality, Vibrancy, and Youthfulness Expert. At 51 years young, she is the living embodiment of her powerful message. As author and creator of *Fit, Fifty & Fabulous… Seven Secrets to the Fountain of Youth!*, she shares her secrets on how to be ageless, timeless, and limitless…and how to always LIVE your heart's desires! www.DrElizabethLambaer.com

Gabriela Volquartz is an actress and a model. www.modelmayhem.com

Jamie Gough is the owner and operator of Simple Site Guru Web Site Design. She is FABULOUS—HIRE HER! *www.SimpleSiteGuru.com*

Dr. Janet Brill is the bestselling author of two books, *Cholesterol Down* and *Prevent a Second Heart Attack*. www.DrJanet.com and www.PreventaSecondHeartAttack.com (Photo credit: Marina Larenz)

Jennifer DiDonato is a personal trainer whose goal is to make the health and fitness goals of all people simple, convenient, and attainable—no matter their condition or fitness level! www.madefittv.com

Jenny Present is a custom jewelry designer specializing in feminine, classic, and unique pieces. www.jennypresent.com (Photo credit: Aime Oberheim, aimelee creative)

Jodean Petersen is a researcher and administrator who is currently employed by a company that owns three separate medical practices including research, organizational, and application divisions.

Joyce Restaino is a writing consultant. Because poor writing creates a negative impression, Joyce helps businesses, organizations, and individuals polish their images through the written word. www.GrowYourBusinessWrite.com

Julie Spira is a bestselling author, dating and relationship expert, social media expert, and serial entrepreneur. www.CyberDatingExpert.com and *SocialMediaMore.com*

Kami Gray is a TV/film wardrobe stylist and bestselling author. She is also a consultant for individuals wanting to improve their styles and update their images. www.kamigray.com

Kathleen Mongero currently practices traditional and new media relations as an account executive at one of Raleigh, North Carolina's top PR firms.

Kathleen Pleasants, owner of Clearly Unique, has been studying and practicing holistic health since 1983. As founder of the World Dance-Fitness Project, she travels the world to bring health and fitness awareness to individuals and their families in many fun ways. www.clearlyunique.net

Kelly Bouchard is happily married with three wonderful grown-up kids. She is particularly passionate about empowering people to believe in themselves and the power of their dreams! www.kellybouchard.com

Kendra Kroll is the creator of PortaPocket strap-onto-the-body carrying cases—the solution to pocket-challenged outfits everywhere, keeping important things safe and comfortably available. www.portapocket.com

Keri Cawthorne is a fitness instructor, avid runner, and writer. She believes that fitness should motivate not intimidate, and prides herself on making her classes reflect that. www.ironmountainmovement.com

Kim McCool travels and teaches portrait painting seminars throughout the country.

Artist, teacher, inspirational speaker, and author, Kim has a passion to share artwork with others. *www.kimmccool.com*

Kim Michelle Richardson is an active community worker doing volunteer work for Habitat for Humanity and a local shelter for the homeless, as well as helping young students with reading and writing. *The Unbreakable Child* is her first book. *www.theunbreakablechild.com* (Photo credit: Andrew Eccles, Andrew Eccles Studio, NY)

Kristi Chrysler is a national speaker, published author, professional certified health coach who inspires others to achieve their maximum wellness potential, and single mother of five! *www.kristichrysler.com*

Kristen Horler developed Baby Boot Camp to balance the fitness needs of new moms, enabling active women to follow their entrepreneurial spirit while spending time with their families. *www.babybootcamp.com*

Lara Dalch is owner of Dalch Wellness, a holistic health counseling practice dedicated to helping busy people balance health, fitness, and lifestyle goals with hectic lives. *www.dalchwellness.com*

Laura Rodriguez is a speaker and writer on awakening the wisdom within that leads to inspiration and innovation for excellence in business and joy in daily life. Her book, *Beginning Yoga for the Non-Athlete: How to Become Slim, Supple, and Serene*, teaches virtually anyone how to feel and look their personal best through the ancient science of yoga. *www.laurasathomeyoga.com* and *www.yogaexercisesforbeginners.com*

Lavinia Rodriguez is a clinical psychologist who specializes in eating and weight problems. She is the author of *Mind Over Fat Matters: Conquering Psychological Barriers to Weight Management. www.FatMatters.com*

Leigh Peterson is in charge of e-marketing for a large music agency, is a professional singer, owns the online pet-lovers gift shop GoFetchGifts.com, and is a VA specializing in copywriting and other Internet-based tasks. *www.LeighVA.com*

Leslie Richin is a freelance journalist, publicist, social media strategist, and event planner. *Twitter.com/LeslieRichin*

Linda Nagamine is an inventor, and founder and president of EZ Living Connection LLC, a privately owned company based in Hawaii. *www.FunKeyFinder.com*

Lindsay Baker is an outpatient oncology dietitian. She enjoys watching reality shows about food and hopes to one day have a show of her own. *www.mcghealth.org* (Photo credit: Pitter Goughnour)

Lisa Blood is a private yoga instructor who teaches everyone from beginners to the seasoned yogi. Her specialty includes personalizing a practice that meets individual fitness and wellness needs. *http://simplepathyoga.wordpress.com*

Lori Brigantino is an actor, writer, and musician who performs regularly in NYC and beyond. She is also a professional copywriter and copyeditor. *www.linkedin.com/in/loribrigantino*

Lori Bumgarner provides image consulting services such as wardrobe edits, wardrobe makeovers, personal shopping, instruction on how to dress your body type, and a variety of career enhancement services for clients who include busy moms, local celebrities, recording artists, and more! *www.paNASHstyle.com*

Lori O'Brien is the president and CEO of a full-service event and entertainment company specializing in corporate events. She is also a vocalist and entertainer. *www.atlantaspecialevents.com*

Lucia is a dating/relationship/media expert, author, radio/TV host, syndicated columnist, and a keynote speaker. *www.theartoflove.net*

Margaret Day is an AFAA-certified group exercise instructor. She is an active mom, an accomplished marketing and sales professional, and student in Bible Study Fellowship International. Fit body, mind, spirit. *www. choosethisday.myarbonne.com* (Photo credit: www.finnigan.photoreflect.com)

Mary Rentoumis is a nutrition enthusiast and author. Want to eat a healthy diet, but can't cook or simply don't have time? Join Mary on her humorous journey to an easy, healthy-eating lifestyle! *www.healthy-diet-mom.com*

Melissa Dinwiddie is a Renaissance woman—artist/designer, freelance writer, and jazz singer/songwriter who inspires people to follow their evolving bliss and live their dreams. *www.melissadinwiddie.com*

Melissa McAllister is a Beachbody Coach. Beachbody is the producer of videos like *P90X* and *Slim in 6* as well as the makers of the revolutionary Shakeology meal-replacement drink. *www.teambeachbody.com/melissamade*

Melody Serafino is a media relations professional and avid freelance writer. She writes for *Time Out New York* and *Examiner.com*, among several other online periodicals. *www.fabulouslyfrugalnyc.blogspot.com*

Merry Lynch is a certified lifestyle expert and etiquette trainer who teaches new levels of effective communication, bringing humor, compassion, patience, and courtesy into play. *www.askmerry.com* (Photo credit: Tracy Kreck of Photographic Passion)

Michelle Mcgough Huffman is the creator and founder of a social networking/e-commerce site tailored for any individual or business who desires success. (Photo credit: ExpectStyle.com)

Monique Caradine is an award-winning producer and host of TV and radio programs. She is also a media strategist, working with high-level executives and entrepreneurs on branding, media messaging, and publicity. *www.MoniqueCaradine.com*

Natasha Drisdelle is a former business development strategist who traded the corporate ladder for Snakes & Ladders to be home with her twin boys. (Photo credit: Shari Rittenhouse)

Nicole Glor is an AFAA-certified personal trainer, group fitness instructor, and fitness columnist for Military.com. She is also the fitness DVD creator of *www.nikkifitness.com*

Nwenna Kai is the author of *The Goddess of Raw Foods*. Her mission is to empower communities around the world to improve their health through a live vegan diet. *www. nwennakai.com*

Patricia Broom is a realtor and owner of a landscaping company. She has been married 27 years and has two beautiful children.

Paula Schafer is a real estate professional. She believes in giving back and is currently on the board of Out Against Abuse—a nonprofit organization that helps victims of domestic violence.

Peg Sausville is author of the e-books *The Truth About How to Kiss Women* and *Thirty Ways to Happier Days,* used to help raise awareness for selected charities/causes. *www.riskhappiness.com*

Rebecca Kussmann is the owner of Bettie Bomb, Inc., a Chicago-based boutique public and media relations agency specializing in lifestyle, nonprofit, retail, fashion, health, restaurant, and hospitality industries. *www. bettiebombpr.com*

Reyna Franco is a New York City based registered dietitian and certified personal trainer. She combines a holistic approach with science-based nutrition and exercise research. *www.reynafranco.com* (Photo credit: Catherine Gibbons)

Sally Shields is an award-winning pianist, composer, speaker, mom, author, radio personality, and home-based biz owner with 21TEN. *www.sallyshields.com*

Shari Fitness is a certified specialist in fitness nutrition, certified personal trainer, and a natural health advocate. She is on a mission to help coach others toward better health and fitness. www.FitTalkNews.com

Sharon Gerdes, a.k.a. "The Dairy Detective," consults with major food corporations to develop healthy products. She writes for several trade publications on bakery, dairy, product development, regulatory, and nutrition topics. dairydetective@att.net

Sharon Gilchrest O'Neill is a marriage and family therapist who helps clients make their relationships the best they can be. She is also an author, family business consultant, and NYC marathoner. www.ashortguidetoahappymarriage.com

Sherri Hagymas is the creator of a money-saving blog that is dedicated to helping readers stretch their dollars and live on less by finding great sales, freebies, and printable retail, grocery, and restaurant coupons, as well as providing scenarios on how to maximize savings. www.luvabargain.com

Skylor Powell received her HHC certification from the Institute for Integrative Nutrition. www.sprouthealthpdx.com

Stephanie Elizabeth is founder of a natural beauty and health blog to help people get and stay beautiful. www.epicbeautyguide.com

Stephanie Larson is the founder of Dancing For Birth™ Prenatal/Postpartum Fitness & Instructor Certification, executive producer of the revolutionary Dancing For Birth™ Fitness & Birth Wisdom DVD, a certified birth doula, childbirth educator, prenatal/postpartum fitness expert, international speaker, and mom of four. www.DancingForBirth.com

Stephanie Mansour, CEO of Step It Up with Steph, is a nationally known holistic health and fitness expert. She's a certified yoga and Pilates instructor, personal trainer, and body image and confidence coach based in Chicago. www.StepItUpwithSteph.com

Susan Armstrong is an expert in profound change. She is an internationally known speaker, award-winning trainer, and author. www.susanarmstrongtraining.com

Suzanne Andrews is the host of Functional Fitness® starring Suzanne Andrews, PBS TV. She is also an occupational therapy practitioner and founder of Healthwise Exercise, specializing in increasing people's functional ability through fitness techniques designed especially for the over-40, plus-size friendly. www.healthwiseexercise.com

Suzanne Duret is an accomplished entrepreneur, business owner, consultant, and author, as well as the creator of an educational business board game and workbook system. www.ShowcasingWomen.com

Suzy Stauffer is the founder of an organization called Beyond the Bus Stop, which encourages and supports women to start nurturing their goals, dreams, and health, and co-author of Women First, Mothers Second. She is also a Beachbody coach who supports busy people to get in the best shape of their lives from home! www.beyondthebusstop.com and www.womenfirstmotherssecond.com and www.youpushplay.com

Tannis Kobrinsky is a certified Pilates and GYROTONIC® instructor. She leads international mind-body retreats and adventures through her business, Health Habitravels. Her DVD is called WELL: worked out with Tannis. www.healthabitravels.com

Teresa Howes is the founder of SkinnyTinis, the brand that plans to revolutionize the way social drinkers think about alcohol and weight management. www.skinnytinis.com

Terri Huggins is a full-time freelance writer specializing in magazine features and blogs related to weddings, beauty, fashion, education, and culture. She also writes various press releases, Web site copy, and brochures for marketing purposes. www.writingbyterri.com (Photo Credit: William Persons of MVP Images)

Terry Roach, M.Ed., registered Kinesiotherapist, is a multi World Masters track cycling champion, motivational speaker, and educator. Her expertise is in body mechanics, fitness education, and functional movements for activities of daily living, work, and sport environments. *www.bodystabilization.com*

Venetia Sheriff worked in the aerospace industry and is now a full-time mother. She is also a swimmer and water-safety instructor for all ages, a volunteer PE teacher at schools for grades K-5. She contributes opinions to various publications regarding nutrition and holistic living.

Victoria L. Dunckley, M.D. is a neuropsychiatrist dually board-certified by the American Board of Psychiatry and Neurology, and the American Academy of Child and Adolescent Psychiatry. She has been in clinical private practice in Orange County, CA, for more than 10 years, and combines nutrition, supplementation, and weight management in her approach to achieving optimal mental health. *www.drdunckley.com/weight-management* (Photo credit: Jody Zorn of Zorn Photography Denver, www.zornphoto.com)

Wendy Battles-Plasse teaches busy men and women how to create a clean-eating lifestyle, free of excessive salt, sugar, and fat, which kick-starts healthy weight loss, prevents disease, and supports aging vibrantly. *www.DontWorryGetHealthy.com*

Wilhelmina Smith is a NYC freelance cellist, as well as founder and artistic director of a chamber music festival on the coast of Maine. *www.saltbaychamberfest.org*

Winnie Anderson creates and executes integrated marketing plans for brick and mortar businesses so owners can focus on what they do best. *www.virtualmarketing-mavens.com*

Ziporah Janowski is the founder and director of Shane Diet Resorts, a weight-loss "camp" for grown-ups that is part of Camp Shane, the longest running children's weight-loss camp in the world. Shane Diet is for young adults and older adults who want to change their lives (and have a cool vacation). *www.shanedietresorts.com*

Also Available by Sally Shields

Free Coaching Available with Sally Shields

If you are in need of support to lose weight, get in shape, change your body or reach your fitness goals, please know that you have my support. I will be your online coach, the same way that someone was there for me, holding you accountable. If I can do it, SO CAN YOU! Give me 90 days, and I'll help you get into your bikini again. Simply visit my website at www.beachbodycoach.com/sallyshields for more info and let this be the year that you achieve your dreams!

Other Books by Sally:

- The Daughter-in-Law Rules: 101 Surefire Ways to Make Friends with Your Mother-in-Law
- The Collaborator Rules: 101 Surefire Ways to Stay Friends with Your Co-Author
- The Speaker Anthology, Vol.1: 101 Stories That Have Inspired and Motivated Audiences from Coast to Coast
- Publicity Secrets Revealed: What Every PR Firm Doesn't Want You to Know

Please visit Sally on the Web at www.sallyshields.com for contests, give-aways, free bonus gifts, Sally's newsletter, blog, 101 Surefire Ways to Market Your Book, Product or Service, free music … and more!

My publisher, Blooming Twig has graciously allowed me to acknowledge my sponsors on the following two pages. —Sally

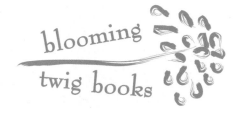

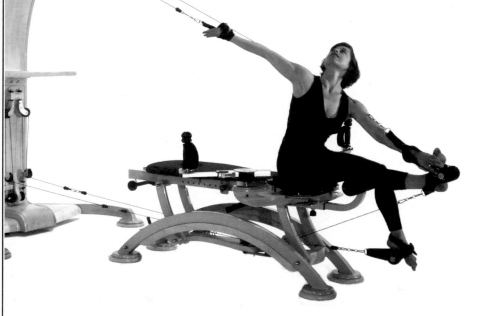

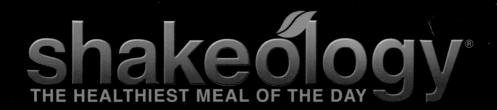

shakeology®
THE HEALTHIEST MEAL OF THE DAY

Nutrition Simplified

70 Healthy Ingredients. 1 Glass.

Why You Need Shakeology® Now!*

Shakeology can help you:

Lose Weight
Feel Energized
Improve Digestion and Regularity
Lower Cholesterol[1]
Tastes delicious, too!

Shakeology Works Two Ways

This patent-pending daily nutritional shake helps your body gently eliminate toxins more efficiently while allowing for better absorption of the essential nutrients you need.*

See What People Are Saying [2]

"I lost 26 pounds."
"I feel more energized."
"My elimination has tripled."
"You look younger."
"My bad cholesterol dropped 57%."
"My favorite thing about Shakeology was the taste."

Independent Beachbody Coach
www.shakeology.com/sallyshields

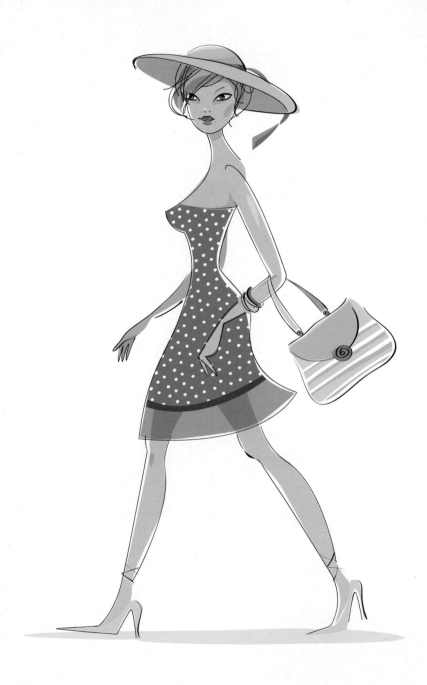